Diabetes

Diabetes

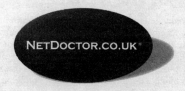

NETDOCTOR.CO.UK®

Series Editor
Dr Dan Rutherford

Hodder & Stoughton
LONDON SYDNEY AUCKLAND

The material in this book is in no way intended to replace professional medical care or attention by a qualified practitioner. The materials in this book cannot and should not be used as a basis for diagnosis or choice of treatment.

Copyright © 2002 by NetDoctor.co.uk
Illustrations copyright © 2002 by Amanda Williams

First published in Great Britain in 2002

The right of NetDoctor.co.uk to be identified as the Author of the Work has been asserted by them in accordance with the Copyright, Designs and Patents Act 1988.

10 9 8 7 6 5 4 3 2 1

British Library Cataloguing in Publication Data
A record for this book is available from the British Library

ISBN 0 340 78684 1

Typeset by Avon Dataset Ltd, Bidford-on-Avon, Warks

Printed and bound in Great Britain by
Bookmarque Ltd., Croydon, Surrey

Hodder & Stoughton
A Division of Hodder Headline Ltd
338 Euston Road
London NW1 3BH
www.madaboutbooks.com

Contents

Foreword

Diabetes is a major and increasing worldwide health problem for all age groups. Globally more than 150 million people have the condition, a figure predicted to exceed 220 million by 2010 and 300 million by 2025. More than 95 per cent of all people with diabetes have the non-insulin dependent form, called Type 2 diabetes. The UK government has now recognised the importance of treating diabetes, with the recent introduction of the National Services Framework for England and Wales and a similar initiative introduced by the Scottish Parliament in 2001.

This book explains in simple terms what diabetes is, describing the different types and their similar end result of elevated blood glucose, which can cause long-term damage to small and large blood vessels in vital organs such as the eyes, the kidneys and the peripheral nerves (so-called microvascular complications) and also to heart, brain and peripheral circulation (so-called macrovascular complications).

Once a diagnosis of diabetes is made, it is important that the diabetic person has the appropriate education and knowledge to manage their condition, whether the treatment is with diet alone, with oral drugs to lower blood glucose or with insulin. What are the principles of diet treatment? What drugs are available and how do they work? Why is insulin necessary and how is it administered and monitored? What is hypoglycaemia (low blood sugar) and how may it be prevented and treated? This book answers these questions and allows the individual to understand diabetes and so more easily enter into partnership with the doctors and nurses responsible for the long-term care of his or her diabetes.

This short text gives an up-to-date review of the current understanding of the practical aspects of diabetes care and gives some insight into the developments that can be anticipated in the coming years.

Professor Ian W. Campbell FRCP, FRCP (Edin & Glasg)
Consultant Physician, Victoria Hospital, Kirkcaldy, Fife
and Honorary Professor, Department of Biological and Medical
Sciences, University of St Andrews, Fife

Acknowledgements

It has been a common experience in producing this book series to find that those colleagues with the least amount of spare time are the most willing to help. Professor Ian Campbell is not only one of the best-known experts on diabetes in the UK but he is also a busy clinician, academic and medical teacher. I very much appreciate Ian's willingness to edit the book in great detail and record time and for his numerous nuggets of information that are otherwise so hard to find. I am also obliged to Jackie Wallace, his secretary, for administrative help.

I am very grateful to my wife, Anne and son, David, who don't see much of me during the writing spells. As always Judith Longman and Julie Hatherall at Hodder & Stoughton have coped with my ever-stretching time demands while still trying to keep to publishing schedules.

Great care is taken to ensure the accuracy of the information presented here and the responsibility for any errors is mine. Please let me know if you spot any, or if you have any suggestions concerning these books. I can be contacted at d.rutherford@netdoctor.co.uk

Dr Dan Rutherford
Medical Director
www.netdoctor.co.uk

Chapter 1

What Is Diabetes?

Diabetes is the condition in which there is a raised level of glucose (sugar) in the blood. The word 'diabetes' comes from the Greek word meaning 'siphon', and refers to one of the characteristic symptoms of the condition – the passage of increased volumes of urine. Diabetes has been known about since antiquity – it is described in the Ebers Papyrus, an Egyptian script dating to 1500 BC – but it was not until the early part of the twentieth century that the cause and treatment of diabetes was discovered.

DIABETES MELLITUS
To be completely correct the term 'diabetes mellitus' should really be used – 'mellitus' is the Latin word for 'honeyed'. There is another diabetes, called diabetes 'insipidus', in which the cause of the increased urine production is a rare hormone disturbance involving the pituitary

gland underneath the brain. Diabetes insipidus is a completely different condition from diabetes mellitus. When people talk about 'diabetes' without any further qualification, they mean diabetes mellitus.

The importance of diabetes

For reasons that we still don't fully understand a raised blood glucose level, if present for years, can cause damage to many tissues such as the eye, kidney and nervous system. Diabetes is the leading cause of blindness and kidney failure in the UK.

Many of the problems arise because high glucose levels damage the fine structure of the arteries throughout the body. Arteries deliver the blood that nourishes every tissue and in diabetes this process is impaired. Diabetes also increases the risk of developing hardening of the arteries (atherosclerosis), which leads to narrowing and blockage of the circulation. The effects of that depend on the organ involved: blockage of heart arteries leads to angina and heart attack, whereas in the brain a stroke can result. These are much commoner in diabetic people.

Fortunately, good treatment of diabetes markedly reduces the chance of serious complications developing. For treatment to be most effective, however, it is important to detect diabetes in its early stages and to treat it right away. A significant proportion of people who are diagnosed with the commonest type of diabetes have had the condition for months or years before it is noticed. That means many already show some signs of diabetic damage before they are even started on treatment.

It is therefore very important that everyone is aware of the possible signs of diabetes and that they are acted upon early. Screening of the population for diabetes has not been done in an efficient or systematic way in the UK (or any other country) and this is a task that we really ought to be doing. However, instead of waiting to be tested in a screening programme an awareness of the symptoms should prompt people to get checked up far sooner than tends to happen at present.

One of the aims of this book is to increase the level of awareness of diabetes in people who might not yet have been diagnosed. The book is intended as an information source for people who are known to have diabetes and for those people who know or care for a diabetic person or who otherwise need to be informed.

That should really include everyone, as diabetes is becoming one of the most important public health problems that we have to face now and in the foreseeable future.

The diabetes 'epidemic'

There are presently over 150 million people worldwide thought to have diabetes and the number is rising quickly – there could be over 220 million affected people by the end of this decade. The fastest rise in numbers is within Western-style populations and is associated with other trends, such as the increasing numbers of people who are overweight, the increasing intake of high calorie foods, fats and sugar and a decreasing tendency of people to take regular and adequate amounts of exercise.

Diabetes is more common with rising age, and develops earlier in some ethnic groups, such as Asians who live in the UK. Perhaps as many as one person in five, over the age of 65 or within these other high-risk groups, has diabetes.

Insulin and the pancreas gland

Diabetes is a complex subject, but one factor is key to the whole issue – insulin. Insulin is a hormone – a substance produced within one part of the body that has its effects in other parts of the body, which it reaches through the bloodstream. There are a great many natural hormones, such as for example the sex hormones that control the production of sperm and eggs or thyroid hormone that controls the body's metabolism.

Insulin is the most important hormone involved in the control of the blood glucose level (although it is not the only one). Blood glucose varies for many reasons – obvious ones being the increase that occurs after a meal or the fall after a long period without food. The extent of these variations in non-diabetic people is, however, quite small. Our in-built correcting mechanisms convert excess glucose into forms suitable for storage and reverse this process when blood sugar is low.

Insulin plays a key part in controlling the reactions of many bodily organs and tissues with glucose. Muscle tissue, for example, will consume glucose for energy when a person is exercising whereas the liver will release glucose from its stores under the same circumstances and insulin makes both of these processes run more efficiently.

The source of all insulin in the body is the pancreas gland – a flattish structure about 15cm long and 5cm wide that lies deep within the abdomen, behind the stomach (see figure 1). The pancreas actually has two functions – one is to produce insulin and the other is to produce a juice that helps us to digest food (mainly fats and proteins). A small tube (duct) connects the pancreas with the upper bowel, just past the outlet of the stomach, and through this duct is released the pancreatic juice. This function of the pancreas is completely separate from the production of insulin – the pancreas is really two organs in one.

Figure 1: Position of the pancreas gland

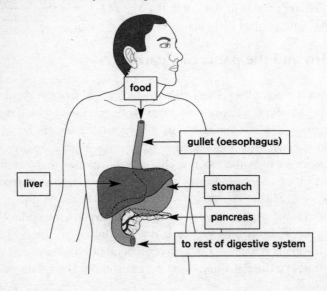

If the pancreas is looked at under the microscope we find there are small clumps of cells, called the 'Islets of Langerhans', scattered throughout the pancreas. (They are named after Paul Langerhans, a German anatomist who first described them in 1869 while still a medical student.) The islets are in fact the hormone-producing part of the pancreas, and all the other cells that surround them are involved in producing digestive juices. More detailed analysis reveals that within the islets there are two main types of cell – the beta cells, which manufacture insulin, and the alpha cells, which manufacture other hormones such as glucagon, whose function we'll come to later (figure 2). Knowing this information about the structure of the pancreas is useful when it comes to understanding the theories of what causes diabetes.

Figure 2: Islets of Langerhans

These are the cells that produce pancreatic juice (used in digesting food).

Islet cells, containing beta cells (producing insulin) and alpha cells (producing glucagon).

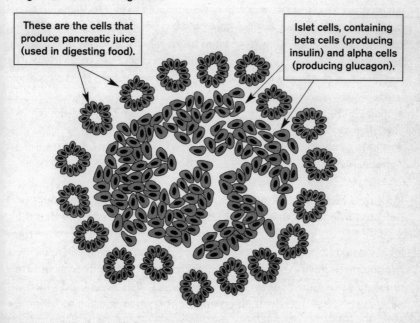

Defining diabetes

Diabetes is about raised blood glucose levels – so what is the normal level? As with any biological measurement this question is not absolutely easy to answer because there is a range of normal values of blood glucose and to some extent the definition of 'normal' and 'abnormal' is artificial. In fact, the level at which blood glucose is deemed too high was re-defined as recently as 1997.

The units of measurement for blood glucose are 'millimoles per litre', meaning millimoles of glucose per litre of blood. This is usually written as mmol/l, or sometimes as mM. To be completely correct it is the concentration of glucose within the plasma of the blood that is actually measured. Plasma is the clear fluid that is left when all the oxygen-carrying red cells are removed from blood. In practice the difference between 'blood' and 'plasma' glucose is unimportant and from now on we will just refer to 'blood glucose' levels.

The definition of diabetes takes into account whether the person having the blood test has recently had something to eat, so there are two categories – one for the 'fasting' state by which it is meant that no calorie-containing foods or liquids have been taken for at least eight hours prior to the test and the second is for 'random' blood glucose measurements taken without reference to when the last food was eaten. The levels are:

- 'Fasting' blood glucose greater than or equal to 7 mmol/l indicates diabetes.
- 'Random' blood glucose greater than or equal to 11.1 mmol/l indicates diabetes.

If a single blood test shows a high reading then of course it should be repeated to confirm that the reading is correct but (assuming that the reading is accurate) if you have a blood glucose that is at or above the levels stated above – you have diabetes. If symptoms of diabetes are present then only one raised blood glucose level is required to confirm the diagnosis. But if there are no symptoms then the blood glucose needs to be confirmed as high on another occasion in order to be sure.

'Borderline' diabetes

Fasting glucose levels below 6.1 mmol/l are normal, i.e. someone with such a glucose level is not diabetic at that point in time. Diabetes can develop at any time in someone's life though, so having a normal reading once does not mean you can never get diabetes.

People who have a fasting glucose level of between 6.1 and 6.9 mmol/l are somewhere in the middle. They are not 'properly' diabetic and do not need specific treatment for their blood glucose level, but they are thought to be at risk of going on to develop full diabetes. This category is called 'impaired fasting glucose'.

'Impaired glucose tolerance' refers to people who have a normal fasting blood level of glucose but whose glucose rises to above 7.8 mmol/l but less than 11.1 mmol/l two hours after taking an oral dose of 75 grams of glucose (this is called a 'glucose tolerance test' and it is explained in the next paragraph). Impaired glucose tolerance (IGT) is more important than just a 'pre-diabetic' state as there is evidence to show that people with IGT are at increased risk of developing some of the conditions associated with diabetes, such as heart disease. People with IGT, in common with those who have diabetes, can improve their outlook by avoiding obesity, increasing their level of exercise and, of course, stopping smoking. They should also be kept under review and checked, at least annually, for the development of diabetes.

Glucose tolerance test

When someone has some or many of the symptoms of diabetes (such as thirst, frequent passage of urine or weight loss) but their blood glucose results have not definitely diagnosed them as having diabetes then a 'glucose tolerance test' can be done. This tests their ability to produce insulin following the oral intake of glucose.

The principle is quite simple – a standard dose (75g) of glucose is swallowed following an overnight fast and two blood samples are taken for glucose measurement. The first sample is taken before the glucose is swallowed, and the second is taken two hours later. If at two hours the blood glucose is 11.1 mmol/l or greater, then the person has diabetes. If the blood glucose is between 7.8 and 11.1 mmol/l then the person has impaired glucose tolerance. If the level at two hours is less than 7.8 mmol/l then diabetes is not present. All of these results are listed in table 1.

Table 1: Diagnosing diabetes – normal and abnormal blood glucose levels (mmol/l)

	Normal range	Diabetic range	'Impaired glucose tolerance'
Fasting	<6.1	≥7.0	<7.0
Random	–	≥11.1	–
Glucose tolerance test (75g glucose given and blood tested 2 hours later)	<7.8	≥11.1	7.8–11.1

Glucose in the urine

That diabetes may be accompanied by glucose in the urine has long been known but it is important to know that glucose does not always appear in the urine of a diabetic person and also that urine can contain glucose despite the absence of diabetes. The reason is because of the way our kidneys work with respect to glucose.

Kidneys are sophisticated filters, allowing the waste products of our metabolism to escape into the urine while conserving other components of blood that are valuable to us, including glucose. Below a certain level of blood glucose (usually about 9 mmol/l) an individual's kidneys will be completely efficient at reclaiming glucose – not a trace will be found in the urine. If, however, the blood glucose goes above this 'threshold' the kidney will start to let some glucose through, and so it will be detectable in the urine. The exact level of the kidney threshold varies slightly from person to person. In some people it is low enough to allow glucose through at normal blood glucose levels. These people do not have diabetes, because it is only the blood glucose that determines whether diabetes exists. Conversely, some people have a naturally high kidney threshold for glucose and show no glucose in the urine despite having high enough blood glucose levels to make them diabetic.

Think of the kidney's behaviour with respect to glucose as being like a harbour wall holding back the tide, where the height of the wall is the kidney threshold and the sea level is the blood glucose. If the wall is high enough then the sea will never cross it – that is the equivalent of our diabetic person with a high kidney glucose threshold. If the wall is built too low, however (equivalent to someone with a naturally low kidney threshold), then seawater will continuously spill over the top (figure 3).

Several points should now be obvious:

- Testing for glucose in the urine is an unreliable way to detect or diagnose diabetes.
- Having glucose in the urine may or may not mean that diabetes is present – further tests are always required.
- Blood glucose measurement is the only way to detect and diagnose diabetes.

Symptoms of diabetes

The blood glucose level, measured under the circumstances outlined above, determines whether someone has diabetes, but what takes a person to his or her doctor is the presence of symptoms of the condition. Perhaps it is more accurate to say that having symptoms of diabetes *should* make someone go to their doctor, as it is well known that many people have diabetes for months or years before it is diagnosed. We will return later to the issue of deliberately looking for diabetes in otherwise apparently healthy people (i.e. population screening).

Figure 3: Role of kidneys in appearance of glucose in urine

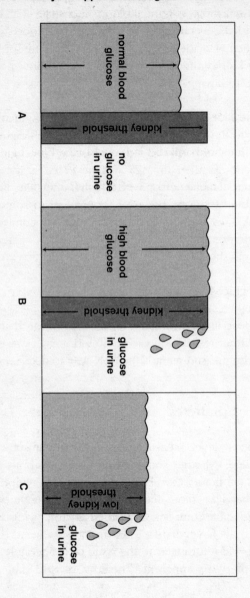

We'll see in chapter 3 that there are two main types of diabetes and the symptoms that are more specific to those types are dealt with there. However, there are several symptoms that are common to all types of diabetes:

- thirst;
- frequent passage of urine ('polyuria');
- fatigue or non-specific ill health;
- blurring of vision (due to changes in the lenses of the eyes);
- tendency to infections (particularly yeast infections like thrush).

You don't need to have all of these symptoms to be diabetic and there are many conditions other than diabetes that can cause the same symptoms. The point is that the presence of any one of them is good enough reason for you to see your doctor and have a check up.

WHAT CAUSES THE SYMPTOMS?
Several of the symptoms result directly from the physical effects of raised blood glucose levels and are due to 'osmosis'. Osmosis is the tendency for water to equalise its concentration when two solutions of different strength are separated by a 'semi-permeable membrane'. A semi-permeable membrane is a barrier whose microscopic structure contains holes large enough to allow through molecules of water, but little or none of the material that's dissolved in the water. For example, if a concentrated sugar solution is placed in a sealed bag made from semi-permeable material and this bag is then immersed in water, water will move into the bag through the pores in the material, making the bag swell. This is because the presence of the sugar molecules makes the sugar solution less concentrated with respect to water. The water outside the bag is therefore drawn into the bag by what is called the osmotic effect.

Figure 4 shows an experiment that can be done in your kitchen if you'd like to prove to yourself that osmosis works!

Figure 4: Osmosis experiment

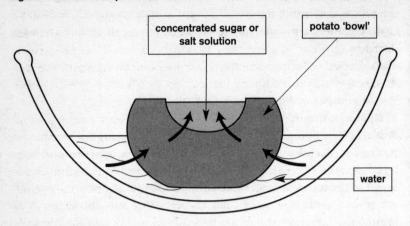

Take a raw potato, peel it and cut it in half. Cut a flat base so it will sit without falling over and scoop out some of the potato so that you have in effect made a small bowl out of the potato flesh. Then sit this potato bowl within a larger, ordinary bowl, and surround it with water to about a third of the way up the side. Then dissolve some salt or sugar in water (enough to make a strong solution) and place this solution within the scooped out part of the potato.

What you have done is create a semi-permeable membrane out of the potato. Each microscopic potato cell is surrounded by a cell wall, which is by far the commonest type of semi-permeable material found in nature. Of course there are actually millions of potato cells in our experiment but as they are all touching each other they act as one. Water in the outside bowl will first be drawn into the potato flesh because there are salts, minerals and sugars dissolved inside the potato cells. Water will also be drawn from the potato into the central well because the solution of salt or sugar you have made will be stronger than the natural concentration of these compounds within the cells. As a result you will see that the level of water within the potato well slowly rises.

It's now possible to explain why a diabetic person can become thirsty and pass lots of urine. If the blood sugar is high enough to exceed the kidney threshold for glucose then we've just seen that this causes glucose to appear in the urine. That urine glucose has an osmotic effect, and draws extra water from the tissues surrounding the millions of tiny tubes that make up the kidneys' filters. Thus the person passes excess amounts of urine, which leads to thirst.

Blurring of vision can be a symptom of diabetes and is also an osmotic effect due to high blood glucose levels acting for months on the lens of each eye. The lens absorbs the extra glucose and then draws in more water from the surrounding tissues. It therefore swells up, which of course changes its optical properties and puts the eye out of focus. A change in spectacle prescription or the development of blurring is therefore one of those other clues to diabetes that we should be aware of.

By the same token, a newly diagnosed diabetic person should put off ordering new spectacles until their blood sugar has been brought back to normal and has stayed that way for at least a few weeks, or else those new glasses will need replacing following the return of the lenses of the eyes to their proper size!

THRUSH

Glucose is an excellent food not just for human beings but also for nearly every other type of living organism, including the yeasts that exist in small numbers even on healthy skin. Some glucose in the urine can be deposited on the genitalia of a diabetic person after they pass urine, so encouraging the growth of yeast and leading to 'thrush' infection – a red itchy irritation of the skin.

Thrush is quite a common problem – more so in women than in men – and many people who do not have diabetes get it too. Anti-thrush cream can now be bought at the pharmacy without a doctor's prescription but obviously it is not wise to keep treating yourself repeatedly if the thrush is not going away – it could mean that you have diabetes. If you are known to have diabetes and are still getting thrush then it probably means that your blood glucose is too high, at least at times, and that your treatment needs to be reviewed.

Non-diabetic people with a low kidney threshold for glucose are prone to thrush and this is most commonly seen in pregnancy, when the mother's kidney threshold will often fall temporarily.

Another clue to the presence of glucose in the urine is the mark it can make if some urine dries out on underpants. Small white crystals of sugar may then be seen.

FATIGUE, MALAISE AND WEIGHT CHANGE

These symptoms relate to the inefficiency or absence of action of insulin within the body, that is part and parcel of diabetes. Insulin is essential for most cells to utilise glucose for energy and without it we easily become fatigued. We also start to burn up reserves of alternative energy such as fat and muscle tissue. Particularly in the type of diabetes that is common in younger people, this can lead to rapid weight loss. Despite the weight loss, appetite is often increased.

This is in contrast with the type of diabetes commoner in older people, which tends to come on more gradually and is usually associated with the person being overweight.

Key Points

- Diabetes mellitus is the condition in which blood glucose rises above normal.
- Diabetes is a major public health problem which is becoming commoner.
- The complications of long-term diabetes can be minimised by good treatment.
- Many people with diabetes are diagnosed late and it is important to recognise and act upon the symptoms of diabetes at an early stage.
- The main symptoms are thirst, frequent need to pass urine, fatigue, tendency to infections, blurring of vision and weight change, but not every symptom will necessarily be present.
- Diabetes is present if the fasting blood glucose level is at or above 7.0 mmol/l, or if the random blood glucose is at or above 11.1 mmol/l.
- A glucose tolerance test indicates diabetes if the blood glucose is at or above 11.1 mmol/l two hours after taking 75g of glucose.

Chapter 2

Energy for Life

When you watch a water wheel turning, it's pretty obvious how it works. You can see the water coming in at the top, striking the paddles and turning the wheel. The driving power comes from gravity – water moves from a higher to a lower position and in doing so gives up its stored 'height energy' to the wheel.

Looking at a living organism does not reveal any such direct link between fuel and function. Knowing that there is a relationship between a bowl of cornflakes and the ability to run for a bus doesn't help to explain how one can be transformed into the other.

Glucose as fuel

For the answer we have to get down to the level of molecules and enter the realm of the biological chemists. The energy that drives life comes from bonds between molecules that are exchanged within the complex reactions that go on in cells. The high-energy molecule that is commonly used in most of these reactions is called ATP. When ATP is changed into a simpler molecule it gives up some of its stored energy, and this is used to power whichever process it is involved in. It is this ATP that is the real fuel that cells need to work – whether it be muscle cells that contract, nerve cells that conduct a signal from the brain or a light-sensitive cell in the retina of the eye.

This is where glucose comes in, because to make ATP in the first place glucose molecules are broken down in a series of steps, each one of which generates a number of ATP molecules.

Carbohydrates

Carbohydrate is the general term for the energy-containing compounds that plants make from carbon dioxide (in the atmosphere) and water (from the soil) in the presence of sunlight and they are the mainstay of the human diet across the world. Glucose is the particular carbohydrate that fuels our energy needs but we do not eat very much in the way of pure glucose. Most of our carbohydrate intake is in other forms, which are then broken down to produce glucose.

There are three major types of carbohydrate as far as foodstuffs are concerned:

- sucrose – the common sugar that we add to drinks and food and which is derived mainly from sugar cane;
- lactose – another sugar present in milk;
- starches – the bulk type of carbohydrate present in grains, rice, potatoes, etc.

Sugars are interesting from the chemical point of view. Sucrose, for example, is in itself a chemical combination of two other types of simpler sugar – glucose and fructose. Lactose is the combination of galactose and glucose. Starches are much larger combinations of many sugar molecules.

Much of the process of digestion consists of breaking down the larger carbohydrate molecules into the smaller types and then ultimately to glucose which we can then convert into energy.

Glucose stores

The importance of glucose to energy provision is therefore easy to appreciate but in its pure form glucose is not stored to any great extent in the body. Instead, molecules of glucose are linked together to form a much larger molecule called glycogen. Glycogen is stored widely in the body, but particularly within muscles and within the liver. When energy is required enzymes within cells chop some of the stored glycogen back into glucose. In the case of muscle cells they can utilise the glycogen stored within them whereas the needs of other tissues are met by the liver, which releases glucose from its stores into the bloodstream, where it circulates to be picked up by any cells that need it.

Both processes – of storage and release of glucose – go on simultaneously and it is the balance between them that determines whether there is a net change in the blood glucose as a result. The liver is the most important organ as far as glycogen stores are concerned, and disturbance in this aspect of the liver's function, as occurs in diabetes, has a marked effect upon blood glucose.

Insulin

We've already covered the fact that insulin is a hormone produced solely by specialised (beta) cells within the pancreas gland. The stimulus to the pancreas that causes it to release insulin is the circulating level of glucose in the blood. After a meal, for example, glucose will rise both because it may be present in food and as a result of being produced by conversion from other foodstuffs by other chemical reactions within the body. This rise in glucose will stimulate the release of insulin, which then has several immediate effects.

First, insulin stimulates the liver and muscle cells to take up glucose and become more active in making glycogen. Second, insulin reduces the liver's output of glucose. These actions reduce the level of blood glucose. Third, insulin activates muscle cells to manufacture protein and fourth, insulin stimulates fatty tissue to take up circulating fat molecules (called fatty acids) from the blood. These actions build up more energy reserves in the body.

Absence of insulin effectively causes the reverse to happen. Blood glucose continues to rise after a meal as there are no correcting influences and the storage of glucose within cells is impaired. Liver output of glucose (from glycogen) carries on at the same rate and circulating fatty acids are not shifted into fat tissues.

INSULIN AND CELLS

Many types of tissue cell, particularly muscles, are unable to take in and use glucose from the blood unless insulin is also present. Figure 5 illustrates why. If we were able to magnify the surface of a single muscle cell and could actually see glucose molecules floating around in the blood we'd notice that glucose does not flow into the cells as a fish swims into a net, but instead there are 'pumps' on the cell that grab glucose molecules and then transfer them into the cell. Insulin molecules are required to activate those pumps, and without insulin they are inactive – glucose just bounces back into the bloodstream. A basic analogy is a revolving door at the entrance to a building. Insulin acts like the key to the door lock. When the key is present, the door is free to rotate and admit glucose to the cell. Take the key away and the door refuses to turn, barring glucose. The real situation is rather more complicated than this, however, as the presence of insulin on the outside of the cell also activates the key processes within the cell that use glucose for energy.

Lack of insulin therefore makes it impossible for these insulin-dependent tissues to use glucose as fuel despite the fact that there is plenty of it circulating in the blood. In the case of muscles what then happens is that they switch to using fat as an energy source. Although this works adequately it has a number of associated problems. First is the fact that the products released by the 'burning' of glucose by cells

Figure 5: Effect of insulin on use of glucose by muscle cells

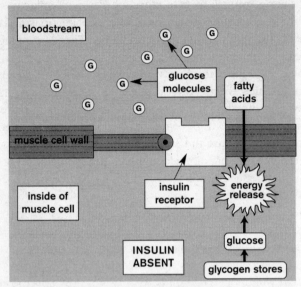

In the absence of insulin, muscle cells use stored glycogen and fatty acids for fuel.

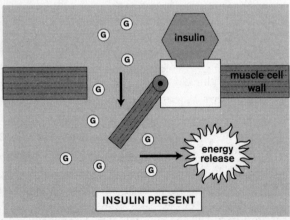

The attachment of insulin to the insulin receptor opens the 'gate' that specifically allows glucose into the cell, and also activates the chemical release of energy from glucose molecules.

are still required for fat to be used efficiently. So energy release is limited – the person still feels tired. Second, a by-product of using so much fat is the production of acids that can have serious consequences for the body's many other chemical processes. These excess acids are called 'ketones' and doctors use the term 'ketotic' to refer to a diabetic person who is producing an excess of ketones. Ketones can have a sweet smell, like acetone, and the presence of ketones on the breath is a characteristic sign of someone with uncontrolled diabetes due to insulin lack.

One of the ways that the body uses to get rid of excess acid is through the breath (breathing out more quickly gets rid of carbon dioxide, which reduces the acidity of the blood), so another common finding in a diabetic person badly needing insulin is that they breathe very quickly.

Diabetic ketoacidosis

This scenario of rising blood sugars and ketone production in the absence of adequate amounts of insulin is called ketoacidosis, or diabetic ketoacidosis (DKA), and it is dangerous. Before the arrival of insulin treatment in the 1920s an episode of DKA would usually be fatal. DKA still happens and it is a medical emergency, but with prompt treatment of the right kind (insulin and fluid replacement) it is usually completely reversible. One of the most important aims of diabetic treatment is the avoidance of ketoacidosis, which really means balancing a person's daily insulin need with the amount that they take.

DKA is a threat only to people whose diabetes is due to absent or insufficient production of insulin, as will be explained in chapter 3.

Glucagon

Up until now the emphasis has been on insulin. Glucagon is the other main hormone produced by the pancreas (it is produced by the alpha cells) and in many ways it is the opposite of insulin. Glucagon acts to increase the blood glucose level, which it does by two actions upon the liver:

- Glucagon increases the rate at which glycogen is converted into glucose for release into the bloodstream.
- Glucagon increases the liver's ability to make glucose from other compounds, such as amino acids. (Amino acids are the 'building blocks' of proteins.)

As with insulin, the most important factor that controls the release of glucagon from the pancreas is the blood glucose level. As blood glucose rises, glucagon output falls and vice versa. Glucagon is released also after a protein meal and after prolonged exercise.

Abnormalities of glucagon production are rare. There is no corresponding condition to diabetes in which lack of glucagon production gives rises to medical problems. It is possible for a tumour of the pancreas to produce excessive amounts of glucagon and cause diabetes but it is extremely rare – fewer than 250 people have ever been described with this condition (glucagonoma) in the world.

Insulin-producing tumours of the pancreas (insulinoma) also exist but again are extremely rare. An insulinoma could potentially cause episodes of low blood glucose every time it released a surge of insulin but by far the commonest cause of low blood sugar is the effect of slightly too much diabetic treatment (see below).

Glucose and the brain

One other point it is important to make concerns the role of glucose as an energy source and how it relates to brain tissue. We've mentioned that muscles need insulin for them to use glucose, but brain tissue does not. Glucose is able to flow freely into brain cells from the blood. The other big difference between brain cells and muscles is that brain does not store glycogen or any other reserve energy source. The brain is therefore completely dependent on receiving a constant supply of glucose from the blood to keep it functioning. If the blood sugar falls the brain will immediately suffer.

If the drop in glucose is slight then the effects may at first be quite mild – a degree of confusion perhaps – although that in itself might be dangerous if, say, it happens while driving a car. If the blood glucose falls further then brain function is progressively affected until unconsciousness results. Provided treatment is given early enough to raise the blood glucose to normal then no lasting damage will result but very low blood glucose levels, if prolonged, can lead to irreversible brain damage.

The medical term for a low blood glucose level is 'hypoglycaemia', or 'hypo' for short. Learning about hypo attacks is part of any diabetic person's education about their disease, and virtually everyone who has diabetes will experience a hypo at some time. More often than not a hypo will be accompanied by some symptoms, which if recognised and acted upon soon enough will stop it getting worse. If the person is still conscious and able to swallow some extra glucose, for example, then that might be all that is needed. When a hypo has led to unconsciousness then help is needed from someone adequately trained to deal with it. An injection of glucagon is one emergency treatment that can work well. If that does not work or it is not available then glucose needs to be injected into a vein.

The reversal of a hypoglycaemic attack, in which a deeply unconscious person can be brought back to full alertness within a minute or two, is one of the most dramatic and gratifying experiences in medicine, but hypos are not desirable from the diabetic person's point of view.

Key Points

- Glucose is a simple sugar and is the main fuel used by living cells.
- Carbohydrates are the foodstuffs from which glucose is obtained by digestion.
- Glycogen is the storage form of glucose and is present in muscle and, especially, the liver.
- Brain cells only use glucose but most other tissues can also use fat and protein as energy sources.
- Brain cells can use glucose directly from the blood but most other tissues require insulin to be present.
- Blood glucose is lowered by insulin and raised by glucagon.
- Diabetic ketoacidosis (DKA) is a potentially dangerous condition caused when insulin lack has led to the excessive breakdown of fatty tissue as an energy source.

Chapter 3

The Types of Diabetes

Type 1 diabetes

In the late nineteenth century it was shown that experimental removal
of the pancreas gland caused dogs to become diabetic. The Canadian
physicians Banting and Best discovered in 1921 that what mattered
was the removal of the source of the hormone that we now call insulin.

Surgical removal of the pancreas is an uncommon operation and a
very unusual cause of diabetes but damage to the pancreas is far
commoner. Today we call this 'Type 1' diabetes. Until very recently
the term 'insulin-dependent diabetes' was used because this type of
diabetes always requires insulin treatment. As will be seen at the end
of this chapter the classification of diabetes is changing in response to
the patterns that we see in the condition worldwide. As this is a recent
change the term 'insulin-dependent diabetes' is likely to be around for
a while yet, but 'Type 1' is the preferred term.

Damage to the pancreas can occur for a variety of reasons such as a viral infection of the gland, but in Type 1 diabetes we now know that by far the commonest cause of the pancreas damage is the body's own immune system. Samples taken from the pancreas of people with Type 1 diabetes show that the beta cells of the Islets of Langerhans have been progressively destroyed by attack from the cells that normally defend us from invading organisms and other foreign material. This is called an 'auto-immune' process, referring to the fact that the body appears to turn against itself in the course of the disease.

There are other auto-immune diseases, such as for example those affecting the thyroid gland, which are seen with increased frequency in people who also have Type 1 diabetes, and this probably reflects an inherited tendency in some people to develop auto-immune disease that is triggered by some other factor in the environment. Exactly what that trigger could be is still unclear but there is some evidence to suggest that a virus infection in such individuals could start the process off. There is also weak evidence to show that the development of Type 1 diabetes is commoner in societies where cows' milk is consumed in larger amounts (see next chapter).

Development of Type 1 diabetes

One of the characteristic features of Type 1 is that it has quite a sudden onset – often just days or weeks during which the typical symptoms become apparent whereas the person prior to that has apparently been healthy. On the surface this is true, but in reality Type 1 diabetes comes on over a much longer timescale. It is only when about 90 per cent of the insulin-producing beta cells are destroyed that the amount of insulin being produced starts to fall below the body's needs.

> **The single process that causes Type 1 diabetes is failure of the pancreas gland to produce insulin.**

Type 2 diabetes

This also has an older alternative name that is being phased out – 'non-insulin-dependent diabetes'. It is far commoner than Type 1 diabetes, accounting for about 90 per cent of diabetic people and it is this type that is becoming so much more common across the globe. People with Type 2 diabetes are usually older than those with Type 1 although the distinction between the two types in all respects, including age, is becoming increasingly blurred. About 5 per cent of middle-aged and older adults within Europe have Type 2 diabetes and in the USA the figure is approaching twice this level.

Type 2 diabetes is strongly associated with being overweight but we are much less clear about what causes Type 2 compared with our understanding of Type 1 disease. In Type 2 diabetes people have high levels of insulin circulating in the blood because the ability of the islet cells to produce the hormone is well preserved (at least until late in the progress of the disease – see below). This is quite different to Type 1, in which the destruction of beta cells and hence falling insulin production occurs early on and is the cause of the condition. However, the *effect* that insulin has on its target tissues (such as muscle and liver cells) is markedly impaired in Type 2 diabetes. So, despite the fact that in early Type 2 there is plenty of insulin available, for reasons that we don't understand the insulin does not switch on the processes of shifting glucose into cells and releasing energy from glucose. This phenomenon is called 'insulin resistance'.

Insulin resistance has a number of important knock-on effects – all off them detrimental to good health unfortunately. Apart from causing high blood glucose, insulin resistance disturbs the fat levels in the blood and makes it more likely for the heart arteries to become clogged (coronary heart disease). Insulin resistance also raises blood pressure and increases people's tendency to develop gout (a painful condition of the joints).

The beta cells (i.e. insulin-producing cells) of the pancreas gland in people with Type 2 diabetes do not seem to undergo the attack from the immune system that is seen in Type 1 disease. Nonetheless the

27

beta cells are unable to cope, for example, with the normal need to produce a surge of insulin after a meal. In people who do not have diabetes this insulin surge stimulates the body to store excess glucose coming in through the digestive system and so keeps the blood glucose level fairly constant. In Type 2 diabetes the inadequate response from the beta cells causes blood glucose to climb even further after meals. This lack of responsiveness from the beta cells is called 'beta cell failure'.

There are therefore two processes going on in Type 2 diabetes:

1 **Inadequate release of insulin in response to raised blood glucose (beta cell failure)**
2 **Inadequate effect of insulin upon the tissues of the body (insulin resistance).**

Type 2 diabetes is therefore quite different to Type 1. In the former there is an excess of insulin production but in the latter there is a deficiency. Type 2 diabetes is a famine in the midst of a feast – there is (initially) plenty of insulin but it becomes increasingly ineffective as time goes on.

The treatment of Type 2 diabetes is covered in more detail in chapter 8 but you can see from the two processes going on in the disease that there are two potential ways to treat it:

- Increase the responsiveness of the beta cells (i.e. make them produce more insulin).
- Reduce insulin resistance (i.e. make the available insulin work better).

These two theoretical ways are indeed the methods used in reality to treat Type 2 diabetes.

Insulin need in Type 2 diabetes

When someone develops Type 1 diabetes they have it forever. As yet we don't have the power to make beta cells work again to produce insulin, so a diabetic person who needs insulin injections due to Type 1 diabetes will always need them.

In Type 2 diabetes, however, the beta cells remain able to produce insulin for many years, although they do so inefficiently. Some of the treatments for Type 2 take advantage of this by stimulating the beta cells to work better but as time goes by there comes a stage in some people with Type 2 diabetes when their beta cells become exhausted. Then, no matter how much treatment is given, it becomes impossible to coax enough insulin out of the pancreas to overcome the person's insulin resistance. Blood glucose begins to climb higher and in effect the person's diabetes has changed into 'insulin-requiring Type 2 disease'.

Often the amount of insulin someone needs in these circumstances is quite large – more than many people with Type 1 diabetes. This is because of the severe insulin resistance people with Type 2 have at this stage of the condition.

Classification of diabetes

In 1997 the American Diabetes Association proposed four types of diabetes, which are now accepted internationally. Type 1 and Type 2 are as already described and are known by those two terms. A third group takes in the various known genetic conditions affecting beta cells as well as other diseases that damage the whole pancreas gland, and the fourth group is that which a woman can develop during pregnancy – called 'gestational diabetes'. For the purpose of this book we'll stick with talking mostly about Type 1 and Type 2. Gestational diabetes is, however, an important subject on its own and is covered in chapter 14.

Type 1 and Type 2 diabetes compared

In chapter 1 the main symptoms that are common to all types of diabetes were mentioned. To remind you, these are:

- thirst;
- frequent passage of urine ('polyuria');
- fatigue or non-specific ill health;
- blurring of vision;
- tendency to infections (particularly yeast infections like thrush).

There are also differences between the diabetic types. The important features that make Type 1 distinct are:

- The disease develops quickly – often over just a few weeks.
- Type 1 diabetes is obvious – it always causes significant symptoms.
- It usually develops in childhood or adolescence (but is also seen in adults).
- Patients tend to be lean.
- Ketoacidosis can occur readily.
- There are antibodies in the blood acting against the pancreas (showing the immune system is attacking the gland).
- Insulin is always needed for treatment (along with attention to diet and exercise).

The particular features of Type 2 are:

- Slower onset – often over years.
- Type 2 diabetes symptoms can be mild and overlooked or ignored for a long time.
- It usually develops in middle age or later.
- Patients tend to be overweight.
- Ketoacidosis occurs only rarely (because some insulin is produced for a long time in Type 2 and this protects against developing DKA).
- There are no antibodies in the blood acting against the pancreas.

- Treatment can vary from diet and exercise only, or be with oral medications as well.

Key Points

- Type 1 diabetes is due to failure of the pancreas gland to produce insulin.
- Type 2 diabetes is due to a) inadequate release of insulin in response to raised blood glucose and b) inadequate effect of insulin upon the tissues of the body.
- Eventually many patients with Type 2 diabetes became unable to produce enough insulin themselves to overcome their insulin resistance, and then need insulin treatment.

Chapter 4

The Causes of Diabetes

This is of course the $64,000 dollar question – 'Why does diabetes happen?' Moreover you may be asking 'Why me?' if you have diabetes.

It should be clear from the preceding chapters that diabetes is not one condition but is several that disturb the production and effect of insulin in the body and lead to a common result of raised blood glucose. The effects of raised blood glucose produce lots of symptoms that are common to all types of diabetes, but in many other respects there are significant differences between the diabetic types, and this applies also to what we think causes them to occur. Some background information on the immune system is helpful at this stage because of its importance in Type 1 diabetes at least.

The immune system

Antibodies are protein molecules produced by the immune system following the entry within the body of foreign material such as bacteria, viruses or toxic compounds. The antibody produced against any invader is unique and remains within the body for years, usually. This is the principle behind immunisation against infectious diseases such as measles or tetanus. Vaccines contain millions of molecules of the organism against which we want to become immune, which have been inactivated in some way so that we don't get the disease itself from the vaccine. However, we do develop antibodies to the organism, which remain, in small numbers, in our blood and the other parts of the immune system (the lymph glands).

If the organism (say, for example, the virus that causes measles) enters the body at a later date it will connect with the measles antibody and remain attached to it. Several reactions within the immune system are then triggered which result in the invader being destroyed. Any material that is 'recognised' and attacked by an antibody is called an 'antigen'.

This process goes awry in auto-immune diseases, in which the immune system turns against natural proteins that are part of some tissue within the body. The presence of antibodies against these tissues can be detected by laboratory tests and indicates that the tissue is under internal attack.

One other element of the immune system is worth a mention and is the 'tissue type' of the individual. On the surfaces of most of our cells there are six proteins called 'HLA antigens'. Each cell in any one individual has the same six antigens but as there are about 150 HLA antigens known the exact combination of any six is unique to each human being (except identical twins, who share the same HLA type). When we hear of the need to find a matching donor for an organ or bone marrow transplant it is the HLA type that people mean. Our HLA type is determined by the genetic information in our cells – the chromosomes.

Type 1 diabetes

The preamble of the last paragraph is because Type 1 diabetes is associated with certain antibodies and HLA types. The antibodies are made against the islet cells, some other proteins associated with the pancreas gland and against insulin molecules too. The HLA types seen in Type 1 diabetes are not unique to the condition but they are twice as common in Type 1 as in the non-diabetic population. Conversely there are some HLA types in which diabetes is virtually never seen, suggesting that depending what HLA type you have, you may be more or less vulnerable to getting Type 1 diabetes.

In about 10 per cent of people with Type 1 diabetes there is some clustering of the condition in that family. The brother or sister of someone with Type 1 disease has a 1 in 16 chance of also developing the condition before the age of 20 compared to the average in the population of 1 in 250. The chance goes up to 1 in 2 if the siblings are identical twins.

These are pointers to the likelihood that some people have a genetic tendency to develop Type 1 diabetes. What then matters is an extra influence from something in the environment that tips the balance towards developing the condition. Three possible groups of trigger factor are currently held to be likely – any one of which might be what makes the difference in an individual's case:

VIRUS INFECTIONS
Viruses rightly get the blame for a lot of human illness, but proving a link between a viral infection and a disease caused by it can be very difficult. One definite association is the infection of an unborn baby with the German measles virus (Rubella). A proportion of these babies are born with Type 1 diabetes – but not all of them, so the link is incomplete. Good evidence linking other virus infections to diabetes is lacking, but the possibility exists that several virus infections can trigger diabetes.

TOXIC SUBSTANCES

The observation that breastfed infants may be less likely to go on to develop diabetes has led to several speculations about milk. These include the idea that some substances present in milk substitutes and baby foods might trigger the immune system to attack the pancreas in later life or that cows' milk might do the same.

A protein present in milk, beta-casein, can cause diabetes in animals. In Iceland, where Type 1 diabetes occurs less commonly than in other Scandinavian countries despite similar genetic backgrounds in the populations, cows' milk consumption is not associated with developing diabetes. This might be because milk from Icelandic dairies has less beta casein compared to Scandinavian cows' milk.

FOOD ADDITIVES

A form of chemical compound that is associated with smoked foods (nitrosamines) is potentially able to damage beta cells.

As with so many diseases, the full facts are not known. For example 5–10 per cent of people with Type 1 diabetes do not have any antibodies against the pancreas cells. Perhaps in them the damage to the islet cells has been more direct and has not come via the immune system. Also the possible causal links to milk consumption, bottle feeding, smoked meat and so on are all largely educated guesswork. Certainly we know that breastfeeding is best for babies, but that does not mean that we should blame bottle feeding if that child goes on to develop diabetes. Nor is there justification for us to get in a panic about drinking milk. We may yet find that there are other, possibly more important, environmental factors involved in causing diabetes that we have not considered so far.

Type 2 diabetes

For a condition that has become three times more common across the world over the past 30 years we are still pretty ignorant about what causes Type 2 diabetes. We know several factors are associated with it:

- obesity;
- family history of diabetes (present in 30 per cent of cases);
- lack of exercise;
- ethnic group (in the UK people of Asian and Afro-Caribbean origin have increased risk of developing diabetes).

We've previously covered the two processes that go on – insulin resistance and beta cell failure. There is some debate among diabetes experts about whether one of these faults develops first and leads to the other but no one is sure. In reality it makes little difference, as both are present in everyone with Type 2 disease.

As far as insulin resistance is concerned, the fault lies somewhere in what happens when the insulin locks on to the receptor protein on the surface of muscle (and other) cells and which normally would then set off the glucose pump and the energy releasing process. The 'knock-on' effects of insulin attaching to the receptor do not happen as they should. There are also some subtle differences in the insulin molecules that are produced in Type 2 diabetes.

We are also in the dark about what causes beta cell failure in Type 2 diabetes. It does not appear to come through the immune system as there are no anti-pancreas antibodies in Type 2 disease.

Genetics definitely play a part as having a family history of Type 2 raises the chances of someone else in the family being affected. If one identical twin has Type 2 then the other twin is 90 per cent likely to have it too. In some populations there is a very high risk of developing Type 2 diabetes – for example the Pima Indians of North America have 50 per cent or more adults affected. However no HLA types are associated with Type 2 diabetes.

The best we can say is that some individuals are genetically likely to develop Type 2 diabetes if exposed to certain other conditions such as obesity and inactivity. This therefore has to be the focus of diabetic treatment, and more importantly, prevention.

Drug-induced diabetes

A small but important number of drugs increase the likelihood of developing Type 2 diabetes. The most common are steroid drugs given either by mouth or injections. Steroids often have to be used this way, for example to relieve a sudden attack of asthma, but such courses of treatment are usually short – a week or two at most – and short courses do not usually give trouble with blood glucose. In conditions in which steroids need to be given for much longer periods of time, such as for example severe rheumatoid arthritis or some of the other 'auto-immune' diseases, then insulin resistance and/or beta cell failure can develop, causing blood glucose to rise. The tendency of steroids to raise the blood sugar goes up with higher doses of the drugs, which is one of the many reasons why the minimum possible dose should be used to obtain the desired effect. (Steroid drugs are also commonly used in inhalers for asthma, but the dose absorbed into the body from this type of treatment is too small to cause significant side effects like diabetes.)

Other drugs well known to raise blood glucose are:

- diuretics (water pills) – commonly used to treat fluid retention and high blood pressure;
- beta-blockers (to a small degree) – commonly used to treat angina and high blood pressure.

In the case of these latter drugs the tendency for the blood glucose to rise is unpredictable. Although diuretics are still widely used and effective for treating high blood pressure the doses used nowadays are lower than was common a decade or two ago, so diabetes (or impaired glucose tolerance) is now a less frequent side effect in that condition. Fluid retention due to failure of the heart's pumping action is, however, treated with more powerful diuretics such as frusemide, which are more likely to disturb the blood glucose.

Most of the time drug-induced diabetes will improve or disappear when the offending medication is withdrawn but someone with a particular tendency to become diabetic might remain so and require treatment for it thereafter. People with Type 1 diabetes can find their blood glucose control is impaired with steroid or diuretic treatment and they may have to increase their insulin dosage accordingly.

Type 1 diabetes does not develop as a side effect of any prescription drug in common use but it can rarely occur through poisoning with toxic chemicals. Vacor is an outmoded rat poison capable of destroying beta cells. Streptozotocin is a drug used experimentally to produce diabetes in animals.

We've now covered quite a lot of the background knowledge necessary to understand what diabetes is and what we think causes it, but before covering the treatments available for diabetes it's worth being clear about what is involved in monitoring the effect of diabetes treatment, as the principles apply to all types and severity of diabetes.

Key Points

- Type 1 diabetes is almost always accompanied by the presence of antibodies to the pancreas gland but these are not present in Type 2.
- In Type 1 and Type 2 diabetes it seems that there is a genetic tendency to develop the condition which then needs a trigger factor (or multiple ones) to make the disease appear.
- Although viruses, toxic substances or food additives are thought to be possible triggers for Type 1 and obesity and lack of exercise for Type 2, the exact causes of diabetes are unknown.
- Some drugs, such as oral steroids, diuretics and beta-blockers can cause or worsen diabetes.

Chapter 5

Monitoring Diabetes

We've seen that in diabetes the blood glucose level is high. Treatment of diabetes aims to keep the blood glucose level as 'normal' as possible and we therefore need ways to measure the effectiveness of the treatment, i.e. the blood glucose level.

Test sticks

Glucose can be easily measured now with a range of chemical tests that are quick and accurate. The commonest and most convenient use coloured test pads stuck to small plastic strips that can be used with urine or blood, depending on the type of stick. Each test pad contains the ingredients for a chemical reaction that needs glucose to take place. When the test pad is dipped in urine or covered with a drop of blood the reaction is set off. After about a minute the colour of the pad changes depending on the concentration of glucose in the sample. To read the result you compare the colour of the pad against a chart or you can put the pad into an electronic gadget that does this for you. Using an electronic meter to read the result is more accurate and gets round any problem that someone might have reading colours if their eyesight is poor or they have colour blindness, for example.

Blood and urine tests

Because it is far easier to obtain a urine sample than a blood sample urine tests have for many years been the main way for many diabetic people to monitor their condition, with blood measurement being used less often. This trend has now been reversed because urine tests are not accurate at reflecting the blood glucose levels.

We covered some of the reasons for this in chapter 1. The kidneys only start to let glucose through to the urine when the blood glucose level is above a certain threshold. In some people that threshold is quite low, so they can show a lot of urine glucose despite blood levels that are not very high. In others the reverse is true, and they might have quite high blood glucose yet show little or nothing in the urine. In pregnancy the mother's kidney threshold for glucose falls and so urine checks give even less idea of the blood glucose. Particularly important is the fact that a urine glucose can only show if the blood glucose level is high (or has been since the last time the person emptied their bladder) – it cannot show when someone's blood glucose is too low (hypoglycaemia). Avoidance of hypo attacks is a very important part of the management of diabetes and blood tests are the only way to detect or confirm them.

Diabetes needs to be well controlled if we are to avoid the complications of the condition as much as possible and urine measurements just don't give the necessary precision required. However, it is worth noting that in certain circumstances urine testing can still be very helpful:

- Some people have very stable diabetes (usually Type 2) that is easy to control and in whom blood tests are regularly within the desirable range and urine tests are negative. They might only need to do blood checks infrequently to confirm that the glucose readings are acceptable and can rely more heavily on urine tests from day to day. If they start to show some positive urine glucose readings (as might occur for example during an illness such as a heavy cold) then the frequency of blood tests can be increased.

- It may be quite difficult for some people to do blood tests very often – perhaps because of frailty, poor eyesight, lack of dexterity or just a dislike of needles. Then urine testing can fill in the gaps in information between blood tests done now and again by a carer or a nurse.

Most of the time, however, we can't get round the fact that blood tests are what's really needed to check how someone with diabetes is getting on with their treatment.

Blood glucose meters

There are now nearly 20 of these electronic devices on the market but they all work pretty much the same way. There are, however, some differences in physical size, type of sticks used, number of readings they can hold in their memory, ability to download readings to a computer and so on, so it is important to ensure that you know exactly how to use your own particular meter. This is something that will be thoroughly explained by the people in the diabetic team – usually the nurse at the regional diabetic centre is an expert in this. Although the meters themselves cannot be prescribed on the National Health Service, the test strips can. Many manufacturers supply their meters free to the diabetic clinic (usually based at a district general hospital), and from that source it should often be possible for a patient to obtain a meter free. The manufacturer will then make a profit from supplying the tests strips, as these are particular to the individual make of machine. Meters that speak the reading are available for people with visual handicap.

All diabetic people who require tablets or injections for their treatment are entitled to receive free prescriptions (for all prescribable items, not just those that are to do with their diabetes), so the cost to the patient of the monitoring equipment should be zero. (People whose diabetes is treated by diet alone have to pay for their prescriptions unless they are exempt for any other reason.)

Finger pricks

Instruments that can measure blood glucose reliably through the skin are not yet widely available, although it will probably not be too long before they are developed. For the moment getting a blood glucose measurement means getting hold of some blood. In common with other creatures, human beings are designed to keep their blood to themselves so the diabetic person has to get used to finger pricks. Specially designed needles (lancets) can be used with spring-loaded devices to make the process easier and much less painful. Lancets are not prescribable on the NHS but again are easily obtained through the diabetic clinic at reduced cost.

HOW OFTEN TO TEST?

This is a very common issue to arise. The answer isn't quite as elusive as the length of the proverbial bit of string, but there is no right or wrong answer. The purpose of glucose checks is to get an accurate picture of how someone's blood glucose behaves during the day (and night), so clearly a spread of results is much more helpful than one taken repeatedly at the same time. Days are different in the amount of activity taken, so the checks need to reflect busy days and quiet days too. When diabetes is newly diagnosed or when medication doses are being changed there can be quite marked fluctuations in the glucose levels, so several blood tests daily may be essential if an accurate picture is to be obtained. In pregnancy a diabetic mother will need frequent daily checks on her blood glucose for example. As is covered later in more detail, modern insulin treatment with multiple doses of short-acting insulin allow the diabetic person to more closely match their treatment against their activities on a day-to-day basis at the expense of needing frequent blood glucose tests. What has to be avoided is the development of an obsession with the blood glucose readings in which endless tests are done in pursuit of perfect blood glucose control – an unachievable goal.

The best regime has to be decided on an individual basis but two or three tests each week before a meal and before bedtime, varying the time chosen to reflect the whole day, will be adequate for the majority of people with stable Type 2 diabetes and many of those with Type 1 as well.

MEASURING 'AVERAGE' GLUCOSE LEVELS

Blood glucose, even in non-diabetic people, is not absolutely steady. It goes up and down according to the time since the last meal and level of physical activity. The variation is wider in diabetes but even when someone's diabetes is well controlled the blood glucose at any one moment of time might be unrepresentative of the general state of someone's diabetic control. What is needed is a measure of the average glucose level over an extended period of time, which will give a better idea if someone's diabetic treatment is adequate.

One way of doing that would be to take hundreds of finger prick tests night and day over several months and then sit down with a calculator and average out the readings. For obvious reasons that is not a method with many points in its favour. Fortunately nature has produced better ways that we can tap into, the commonest of which is to measure something in the blood called glycated (or glycosylated) haemoglobin.

Glycated haemoglobin

Haemoglobin is the protein molecule that is present in every red blood cell and which has the job of transporting oxygen in the blood. Haemoglobin locks on to oxygen molecules from the air we breathe as red cells pass through the lungs. Out in the tissues of the body oxygen gets used up and when a red blood cell flows through this area its haemoglobin molecules release their oxygen load.

Glucose in the blood reacts slowly with haemoglobin to form a stable compound called glycated haemoglobin, which is known by the abbreviation 'HbA$_{1c}$'. The amount of HbA$_{1c}$ formed depends on the average glucose level in the blood and because it is formed very slowly it reflects the average blood glucose over the preceding six to eight weeks. In non-diabetic people the amount of HbA$_{1c}$ is about 6 per cent of the total haemoglobin. This is the target to aim for when tight blood glucose control is desirable, although a level of 7 per cent or less is acceptable. Increase in the HbA$_{1c}$ level indicates poorer diabetic control with consequently increased risk of developing the long-term complications of diabetes. The United Kingdom Prospective Diabetes Study Group (UKPDS) was a 20-year long research trial in diabetes (see appendix A) which showed that for every 1 per cent rise in HbA$_{1c}$ a Type 2 diabetic person is 30 per cent more likely to develop those complications arising from damage to the small blood vessels of the body (see chapter 10). In Type 1 diabetes the same relationship between high HbA$_{1c}$ and increased development of complications was shown by the Diabetes Control and Complications Trial in the USA. HbA$_{1c}$ above 7.5 per cent shows only fair control of diabetes and above 8.5 per cent poor control.

Key Points

- Urine tests for glucose are not sufficiently accurate for monitoring diabetes but they can give useful additional information in some people.
- Blood glucose measurements are essential to accurately assess blood glucose control and in particular to detect hypoglycaemic attacks.
- Equipment to measure blood glucose is available free or at low cost to people with diabetes.

- The HbA$_{1c}$ level is a blood test that reflects the average blood glucose level over the preceding six to eight weeks.
- The HbA$_{1c}$ level is strongly related to the likelihood of developing long term diabetic complications and should be consistently kept below 7 per cent if possible.

Chapter 6

Treatment of Diabetes – General Aspects

There are many differences in the treatments for Type 1 and Type 2 diabetes, which are covered in chapters 7 and 8 respectively, but there are also many similarities and we cover these here.

The treatment of diabetes can seem far more complicated than it needs to be and much of any possible confusion can be eliminated by bearing in mind a few basic principles:

- The aim of diabetic treatment is to keep the blood glucose as normal as possible.
- Insulin lack, directly or indirectly, is the basis of diabetes.
- Insulin moves excess glucose into storage (in the liver) and moves glucose into muscles for use in activity.
- The amount of energy the muscles need depends on the person's level of activity.

If one spends a bit of time thinking about what this all means then it becomes obvious that:

- Food intake (energy intake) needs to be balanced against activity (energy output).
- Insulin is required for both of these functions.
- In both Type 1 and Type 2 diabetes, therefore, the common need is for *diet* and *exercise* to be matched.

Cardiovascular risk

Before we move to covering specific areas one other very important point needs to be made concerning diabetes in general, and that is in connection with what's known as 'cardiovascular risk'.

'Cardiovascular' means the heart and circulation, diseases of which are common in western society. These are angina, heart attacks and associated conditions involving 'hardening of the arteries' throughout the body. The UK has one of the worst records in the world for cardiovascular disease. This is for many reasons, including our high-fat diet, tendency to eat lots of salt (which raises blood pressure) and to take inadequate amounts of exercise as well as the effect of smoking. Diabetes increases the risk of developing cardiovascular diseases by as much as four or five times, which is why it is so important not only to treat diabetes well, but also to tackle the other factors that have an influence on the chance of someone developing cardiovascular disease – otherwise called the 'cardiovascular risk'. The most important cardiovascular risk factors apart from diabetes are:

- smoking;
- raised blood pressure;
- raised blood fat (lipid) levels – mainly cholesterol and triglyceride;
- excess body weight.

Blood pressure is dealt with elsewhere in this book, but in summary it should be equal to or better than 140/80 mmHg in diabetes.

The two main fats in the blood are cholesterol and triglyceride. It is clear from many studies that lowering cholesterol to below 5 mmol/litre reduces the risk of cardiovascular disease but the effect of reducing raised triglyceride has been more difficult to prove. Evidence on the effect of triglyceride lowering in diabetes is the subject of current medical research, so as yet the level of triglyceride that should be aimed for in diabetes has not been precisely decided. In the meantime one should concentrate on getting the total cholesterol level down to within the desirable range. In practical terms, the dietary changes that improve the blood cholesterol level will also lower raised triglyceride levels.

Body weight

Excess body weight is associated with high blood pressure, Type 2 diabetes and increased risk of cardiovascular disease. Weight and height are related and knowledge of both is needed before one can say if a person is overweight. A simple mathematical formula relating the two is now universally used to do this – the Body Mass Index (BMI). To calculate a BMI, take the person's weight (in kilograms) and divide it by the square of their height (in metres). For example an 80kg person of height 1.7m will have a BMI of $80/(1.7 \times 1.7) = 27.7 \text{ kg/m}^2$ (the BMI formula applies equally to men and women).

The ranges of BMI are:

- Normal   = 20–24.9
- Overweight = 25–30
- Obese   = Over 30

Table 2 shows a range of heights and the associated weights for the normal and obese ranges. In all people it should be the aim to achieve a BMI within the normal range. Diabetes is much easier to control when the BMI is normal – many people with Type 2 diabetes find that the condition disappears if they get their weight down to the desired level.

Table 2: Body mass index guide

Height (less shoes)			Weight range (kg)	Obese weight (kg)
Metres	Feet	Inches	for BMI 20–24.9	for BMI >30
1.50	4	11	45–56	68
1.52	5	0	46–58	69
1.54	5	1	47–59	71
1.56	5	1	49–61	73
1.58	5	2	50-62	75
1.60	5	3	51–64	77
1.62	5	4	52–66	79
1.64	5	5	53–67	81
1.66	5	5	55–69	83
1.68	5	6	56–71	85
1.70	5	7	58-72	87
1.72	5	8	59-74	89
1.74	5	8	61-76	91
1.76	5	9	62-77	93
1.78	5	10	63-79	95
1.80	5	11	65-81	97
1.82	6	0	66-83	99
1.84	6	0	68-85	102
1.86	6	1	69-86	104
1.88	6	2	71-88	106
1.90	6	3	72-90	108

Diet

Huge amounts of information have been written on diet in diabetes, to the extent that it can all seem a bit daunting and bewildering, yet any such confusion is unnecessary.

> **There is no difference between a diabetic diet and a normal healthy diet that everyone ought to follow.**

There is a common myth that diabetic people need to 'watch their calories' compared to 'healthy' people. This is only partly correct. Everyone's calorie intake should be appropriate for their level of activity, whether or not they have diabetes. The difference between people who do and do not have diabetes is that those without diabetes still have the capacity to overcome excesses in their diet by producing extra insulin to maintain the blood glucose at a normal level. But that does not mean to say that a non-diabetic person can freely take whatever they like to eat and disregard the consequences. Eating less than you need means that you will lose weight and eating more means that you will become overweight – it is not rocket science.

The principles of healthy eating in diabetes are:

- **Eat regular meals.** Starchy foods such as potatoes, pasta, bread, rice and cereals release their energy slowly as they need to be digested first. Therefore they do not cause high surges of glucose in the blood in the same way as sugary foods do.
- **Cut down on high sugar foods.** Foods with sugar (sucrose or glucose) require little or no digestion for the sugars to be absorbed and so they cause blood glucose to rise quickly after a meal. A non-diabetic person can produce the insulin boost to cope with that, but a diabetic cannot. 'Diet' drinks contain sweeteners that have hardly any calories and are a good alternative for those who like sweet drinks. Ignore 'diabetic' foods if you see them. There is nothing special about them, they are more expensive and some actually contain more fat than ordinary brands.
- **Reduce the amount of fat in the diet.** Weight for weight fat has the most calories so cutting down fat intake is an easy way to reduce the total amount of calories eaten. Reducing fat intake (especially hard fats from animal origin) is an essential part of reducing raised

cholesterol and lowering the chance of getting heart disease. Low fat choices are now easy to find in supermarkets, and by grilling, steaming or microwaving foods you can avoid adding fat during the cooking process.

- **Eat five portions of fruit and vegetables daily.** A good intake of fruit and vegetables is proved to reduce blood pressure and protect against many other conditions including heart disease and probably some cancers as well as providing the essential vitamins and minerals we all need.
- **Cut down salt intake.** The recommended total daily intake of salt for adults is 5 grams or less – a slightly heaped teaspoonful. Common salt is sodium chloride and the sodium content of food may be marked as grams or as millimoles (mmol). The conversion is approximately 17 mmol per gram – so you are looking to get your daily intake to below 85 mmol of sodium. That amount has to include all the 'hidden' salt in processed and packaged foods, so it leaves little room for the addition of salt at the table or in cooking. We can easily take two to five times as much salt as we need without trying because so much unnecessary salt comes to us in every variety of food – a single slice of bread can contain 0.5g of salt. It is worth noting how much sodium is present in what you buy and starting to look for lower salt brands. They are beginning to appear in greater numbers on supermarket shelves as the message begins to get through to the food industry that we want less salt.
- **Alcohol.** Consuming a small amount of alcohol daily (up to two standard units) appears to have a beneficial effect upon cardio-vascular risk. There are many possible explanations for this, but among the most likely are that compounds within some alcoholic drinks, particularly red wine, mop up 'free radical' molecules that are capable of causing tissue damage. However, the effects rapidly turn from beneficial to harmful when higher levels of alcohol are consumed. In diabetes alcohol can lower the blood glucose level and therefore make it more likely for a hypoglycaemic reaction to occur. Drinking on an empty stomach makes a hypo more likely too, so it should be avoided.

The usual recommended maximum consumption of alcohol per week for diabetic people is:

- 14 units per week for women;
- 21 units per week for men.

A unit of alcohol is:

- 250ml (1/2 pint) of ordinary strength beer / lager;
- 1 glass (125ml / 4 fl oz) of wine;
- 1 pub measure of sherry / vermouth (1.5oz);
- 1 pub measure of spirits (1.5oz).

DIETARY ADVICE AND CARBOHYDRATES

Because diabetes is about glucose control and glucose is a carbohydrate a lot of the dietary advice that used to be given out in diabetes was about the amount and timing of the carbohydrate intake. Carbohydrate foods were allocated a value per portion – the 'exchange' – and a diabetic diet was constructed around the number of exchanges of carbohydrate that it contained. For example a small thin slice of wholemeal bread contains 10 grams of carbohydrate and is one portion, or exchange, and an individual might be on '200g carbohydrate', which would contain 20 exchanges in the whole day.

Although it will always be necessary to be aware of what you are eating modern thinking has moved away from this type of diet, for various reasons. First is the obvious one that all foods have an energy value, not just carbohydrate. Protein and fat are partly converted to glucose in the body, so they need also to be taken account of. Second is the fact that carbohydrates vary in the rate at which they affect the blood glucose. Pure glucose is absorbed very quickly and within minutes causes blood glucose to rise. Starchy foods, although also carbohydrate, are absorbed much more slowly and they elevate the blood glucose over a longer period of time (see next paragraph). Third is the need to keep the balance within a diabetic diet just the same as a non-diabetic one and basing the diet only on the carbohydrate intake does not do that.

Glycaemic index

This is a grading system that sorts carbohydrates into groups according to the speed with which they elevate blood glucose. Pure glucose has the highest glycaemic index and other foods in the same category include honey, sugar-coated breakfast cereals and sugary biscuits. Foods with a low glycaemic index include brown rice, pasta, porridge, apples, etc. Avoiding swings in blood glucose is easier by choosing foods with a low glycaemic index, but as always a balance between the different carbohydrates is best. Equally it is unnecessary to become obsessed with such a system. It is usually pretty obvious which foods have a lot of sugar in them and a simple rule is to keep them to the minimum.

Dietary advice in diabetes needs to be tailored to the individual and it is impossible to cover anything other than the general points in a book like this. Every diabetic person should have access to a qualified dietician through their GP or diabetic clinic and should make good use of their advice. The dietician will help you work out what your daily calorie needs will be, taking into account your age, lifestyle, work, activities and other points including ethnic diets. She will identify any problems with your diet and be available for advice if you are having difficulties. Most of all she will help you understand the relationship between what you eat and what you need, because once you have understood that then the diet aspect of your diabetes will fall easily into place.

In addition to the information you can get from the dietician there is a wealth of excellent material from diabetes support organisations such as Diabetes UK. Contact details are in appendix C.

Exercise

The other main aspect of treating diabetes of all types is exercise. Food is our energy source and if we compare it with a petrol engine then insulin is the oil that makes all the component parts run efficiently. The fact that Type 2 diabetes is increasingly common appears to be strongly related to increasing numbers of people who are overweight, and in turn this is associated with the fall in popularity of taking exercise. Compared with our predecessors of just 50 years ago we are pretty inactive. We take cars for journeys of a few hundred yards, or sit in trains for hours commuting and spend huge amounts of time at desks, watching TV or otherwise not burning up much energy. For the vast majority of us gathering food no longer means having to work a plot of land but instead is a walk along the aisles of the local supermarket. Taking exercise is a lot more hassle than taking none and unfortunately we are reaping the problems that this brings.

It's perhaps a good place here though to say that diabetes should not be regarded as the inevitable lot of anyone who puts on weight and/or is sedentary. Within the causes of Type 1 diabetes, for example, a lack of exercise is unimportant and 30 per cent of people with Type 2 diabetes are not overweight. So even if we turned overnight into a nation of fitness addicts, diabetes would not go away.

What is clear though is that regular exercise can vastly improve the control of diabetes, and this is particularly true of Type 2.

HOW DOES EXERCISE IMPROVE DIABETES?

Several processes are involved in this, and muscles are particularly important. Muscle makes up a substantial proportion of the body as a whole and, as was seen in chapter 2, muscles need insulin in order to take up glucose from the blood. In the absence of insulin muscles use fat as an alternative energy source, which leads to acidosis if it goes on too long. So insulin allows muscles to burn energy more efficiently and thereby prevent excess calories from being laid down as fat. Diabetes treatment makes insulin more available – either through insulin injections (Type 1) or through the effect of oral medications (Type 2). Increasing exercise usually helps weight loss, which is the other main way that it improves Type 2 diabetes. Thus there is a co-operative effect between exercise and diabetes improvement.

The effect of exercise on glucose control is however quite complex and one of the more problematic areas that needs to be understood by people with Type 1 diabetes is covered in chapter 7.

BENEFITS OF EXERCISE

There are many benefits to exercise for a diabetic person – these are some:

- lower blood glucose levels during and after exercise;
- less insulin resistance;
- lowering of 'bad' cholesterol (low density lipoproteins) and elevation of 'good' cholesterol (high density lipoproteins);
- lowering of blood pressure;
- increased fat loss;
- aid to weight loss;
- increased muscle mass;
- reduced stress and improved well-being;
- improved circulation and reduced cardiovascular risk.

These are substantial benefits for very little outlay. Against the tide of rising numbers of people with diabetes exercise is one of the most important weapons.

HOW MUCH IS ENOUGH EXERCISE?

Surprisingly little, is the short answer. A brisk walk of 30 to 40 minutes taken at least three times a week is enough to improve someone's fitness level and significantly reduce their cardiovascular risk. A diabetic person is looking to do more than this because there is a daily need to 'balance the budget' of the amount of energy taken in and that used, if one is to avoid putting on weight. A daily walk is therefore the ideal amount to be aimed for and five days out of seven is the minimum. There are many ways of achieving this. Using stairs instead of a lift, cycling rather than using the car for short journeys, getting off the bus or tube a stop early and walking the rest can all help to make exercise part of the day rather than an add-on extra. Delegating exercise to something that is done only at a certain time or in a particular place like a fitness centre makes it likely that, as often as not, it won't happen. It is also necessary to spread activity across the day to help keep the blood glucose level steady for as much of the time as possible.

Getting started on an exercise plan can be quite hard, especially if you've been out of the habit for a while. People who are over 40 or are unsure about their suitability to take up exercise should discuss the matter first with their doctor, but the vast majority of people can take regular exercise at a level that benefits them. At first it might mean only a five-minute walk, building it up by a couple of minutes a week.

Hard enough exercise is when there is a feeling of working quite hard but being still able to talk during it. Attention should be paid to building up to a maximum pace and then slowing down before the end of the session. If walking or jogging then good footwear is essential. Try to take a walk where there is some enjoyment from the surroundings, if possible. If exercise is made to be fun then it is a lot more likely to get done on a regular basis.

Lifestyle

Diet and exercise are the basic components of 'lifestyle intervention' for diabetes. Not only are they essential parts of diabetic treatment but also there is good evidence to show that they can delay the onset of Type 2 diabetes. A large study carried out in the USA by the Diabetes Prevention Group observed over 3000 Americans whose blood glucose levels were elevated but below the threshold required for diabetes to be diagnosed. The participants were split into three groups – one of which was observed but given no treatment, another was given a drug (metformin) that lowers blood glucose and is a standard treatment of

Type 2 diabetes and the third group was assigned to lifestyle intervention. The latter meant a goal of 7 per cent weight loss and at least 150 minutes of physical activity per week. Over an observation period of just under three years the people who were given lifestyle intervention had less than half the occurrence of Type 2 diabetes compared with the group that were simply observed. They also had significantly better results than the drug-treated group.

Key Points

- Diet and exercise (lifestyle modification) are essential parts of diabetic treatment.
- Lifestyle modification can delay, and perhaps prevent, the onset of Type 2 diabetes.
- The basic elements of a healthy diet are the same in diabetic and non-diabetic people.
- Exercise improves diabetes and most other risk factors for cardiovascular disease.
- The amount of exercise that is beneficial is the equivalent of a brisk walk for 30 or more minutes on most days of the week.

Chapter 7

Treatment of Type 1 Diabetes

Basic principles

Someone with Type 1 diabetes lacks the ability to produce insulin from his or her pancreas gland; hence the basic treatment is to supply the missing hormone. Insulin is a large protein molecule and it is destroyed by the action of stomach acid and the digestive enzymes of the gut, so it cannot be given in oral form – all insulin needs to be given by injection. The healthy pancreas gland releases insulin according to the level of blood glucose, which varies most according to the intake of food. The aim of the diabetic person is to mimic the natural release of insulin through the timing of their injections and by using a combination of insulin preparations that are absorbed at different rates (figure 6).

Despite the huge efforts that have gone into diabetic treatment over the past 50 or so years we still do not have the perfect insulin delivery

Figure 6: Normal release of insulin during the day

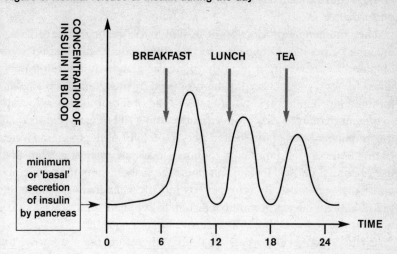

system. What we do have are different preparations of insulin and injection devices that allow choice and flexibility in insulin treatment. With enough time, information, practice and encouragement it is possible for a Type 1 diabetic person to get close to copying nature and maintain good blood glucose control but at the start the process can seem quite daunting. Many health professionals, including doctors, also feel somewhat intimidated by Type 1 diabetes in particular as there seems to be so much that one needs to know – different insulins and injection devices, timings of injections and how much to give when, etc. One of the aims of this chapter is to de-mystify insulin treatment, because it really is quite a simple process.

Insulin preparations

When insulin treatment was first introduced in the early part of the twentieth century its effect was profound. What was previously an extremely serious disease with a fatal outlook suddenly became treatable. Modern diabetic treatment can allow patients to lead a virtually unrestricted life, including those at the very top of athletic performance.

The commercial production of insulin made treatment available to millions of people. Originally (and to some extent still) insulin was obtained by extracting it from the pancreas glands of cows and pigs killed for food production. Insulin produced by these animals is similar to human insulin but it is not identical. One of the problems with any treatment that involves a product made from a different species is that the immune system of the treated person recognises the foreign nature of the treatment, and therefore mounts a response against it. Thus the use of animal-derived insulin can cause the diabetic person to develop antibodies against it. By removing as much contaminating protein as possible the tendency for animal insulin to stimulate antibody production can be reduced, but not to zero.

In the past several years there has therefore been a move to producing insulin by different means that a) are not dependent upon animal sources and b) do not cause reactions within the immune system of the patient. Gene technology has made this possible.

The basic structure of all proteins (of which insulin is only one) is a chain of amino acids linked together – what makes proteins distinct is the number and sequence of the amino acids that they contain. The information that determines these amino acid sequences is held within our DNA – the genetic code that is present within every living cell. Scientists have isolated the section of DNA that codes for the production of insulin and have inserted this gene into the DNA of bacteria and yeasts. These modified organisms go about making copies of the proteins that are coded for by their own DNA as normal but they also churn out copies of insulin in the process. This insulin is extracted and made into an injectable form for use by patients. There are other ways to make human-type insulin such as by modifying pig insulin. The result is insulin that is identical to the naturally produced human hormone and also the elimination of the need to remove foreign proteins.

Everyone who now develops Type 1 diabetes will be treated with 'human' insulin, but there are large numbers of people who were started on animal insulins and have been very well controlled on them. Drug manufacturers still make animal insulins and will continue to do so for some years yet, but it is likely that over the next decade or so animal insulins will be completely phased out. There is however no immediate need for someone using animal insulins to convert to human insulin.

All insulins are now produced to a standard strength – 100 units of activity per millilitre of volume, usually written as '100 U/ml'.

CONTROLLING INSULIN ABSORPTION

Until someone comes along with a device that painlessly and conveniently can continuously monitor blood glucose and then release exactly the right amount of insulin required at any given time we have to rely upon techniques that copy the patterns of insulin release by the body. The main factor that causes insulin to be released is of course the blood glucose level, which goes up after eating food. One way of giving insulin is therefore to inject some shortly before a meal – during the time that the meal is being digested and absorbed the insulin will be taken up by the bloodstream from the injection site. This is a common method used by many millions of diabetic people throughout the world and allows a lot of flexibility – for example if the meal is delayed a bit then the injection can be postponed to suit.

Such a regime of injections does however require that the insulin is absorbed quite soon after being injected, which leads us to an important aspect of insulin treatment – control of the speed of insulin absorption. It was found quite early on in the history of insulin treatment that some chemical tricks could be applied to insulin that would slow up the rate at which it would be absorbed from the injection site. Two substances – zinc and a simple protein called protamine – were found to be useful in this regard and they remain so today.

In the presence of zinc or protamine, insulin molecules gather into larger groups. These groups, although still extremely small, are too large to be absorbed but they slowly break apart, releasing individual insulin molecules that are then taken up by the bloodstream and travel round the body to the various tissues where insulin has its effects. Zinc slows the absorption more than protamine. Although it is possible to use both protamine and zinc together this type of insulin is now less commonly used – insulin combined with *either* zinc or protamine are the types now commonly in use.

The combination of insulin with protamine is commonly called 'isophane' insulin (sometimes written down as 'NPH' insulin).

SITES FOR INJECTIONS

Figure 7 shows the preferred sites for injecting insulin, which are the lower tummy, upper outer arms and thighs and buttocks. It is important to regularly change the injection site – overuse of one area causes the fatty tissues there to either thicken (common) or become thinner (uncommon), both of which can lead to erratic absorption of the insulin from that injection site. This change has the medical name of 'lipo-dystrophy', or 'lipos' for short. Lipos can't always be completely avoided but they are much less likely if injection sites are rotated and injection needles are not re-used too much.

The technique of carrying out the injection is something that is taught by the members of the diabetic team – usually the diabetic nurse. The aim is to get the insulin within the fatty layer under the skin but not too deep so that it goes into the muscles. There are several lengths of needle and techniques available that can ensure this is easy to do repeatedly.

QUICK AND SLOW ACTING INSULINS

These are the two main groups of insulin in use. Quick acting insulin is very soluble, is fairly rapidly absorbed from the injection site and is easy to recognise, as it is always a clear solution in the bottle or cartridge in which it is supplied. Slow acting insulins are those that have been combined with zinc or protamine to slow their rate of absorption and because of that they are always cloudy in the bottle. In

Figure 7: Preferred injection sites for insulin

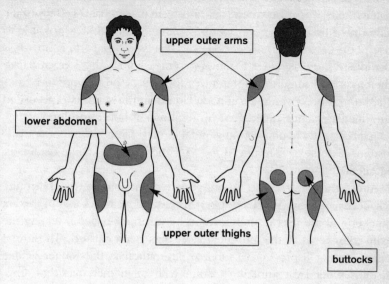

fact 'clear' and 'cloudy' insulins are often how people refer to them. (There is an exception – insulin glargine is a new long-acting insulin made by Aventis and available in the UK from August 2002. It is the first clear long-acting insulin.)

Combining clear and cloudy insulins in different ways to cover the needs of a Type 1 diabetic person is the basis of insulin treatment. Everything else, to do with human or animal insulins, the names given to various insulin mixtures by different drug manufacturers and the different injection devices, etc. are all secondary aspects – we'll be covering them shortly – but if managing Type 1 diabetes ever seems to be getting complicated it does no harm to remember this basic principle.

ACTION TIMES OF INSULINS

- Soluble (clear) insulin starts working 30 to 60 minutes following injection under the skin, peaks at two to four hours and in total lasts six to eight hours.

- Longer acting (cloudy) insulins take one to three hours to work, have most effect between four and twelve hours and last up to 24 hours or more.

Obviously there is quite a range of times within the longer-acting insulins, because of the different properties of protamine and zinc. Therefore it is convenient to divide cloudy insulins into two groups – 'intermediate acting' which last up to about 12 hours and long acting which last 18–24 hours. An old general term still in use for intermediate insulins is 'lente' (pronounced *len-tay*) and for long acting insulins is 'ultralente'.

Although there used to be only one type of soluble (quick-acting) insulin two other types have been recently developed that are even quicker and are useful, therefore, to be given soon before eating, or even afterwards if the pre-meal dose has been missed. These are called insulin lispro and insulin aspart. Whereas the longer acting insulins work by combining insulin with other materials that slow down the absorption, these very quick-acting insulins have been developed by slightly changing the insulin molecule itself. Another term used for them is 'insulin analogues'. The different timescales of the various insulin preparations are shown in figure 8.

Insulin treatment involves combining short and longer acting types and exactly which combinations will suit any individual requires skill and experience to judge. It is one of the jobs of the diabetic specialist, along with the GP and other involved members of the health care team to make that judgement initially but also to help the diabetic person gain sufficient understanding of their condition so that they can learn to make adjustments themselves to their dosage and diet to cope with daily life.

INSULINS IN CURRENT USE

There are four main manufacturers of insulins and someone with Type 1 diabetes should be able to stick with one manufacturer's products. It is therefore unnecessary to know all about the different brands but it

Figure 8: Timescales of action of different insulin preparations

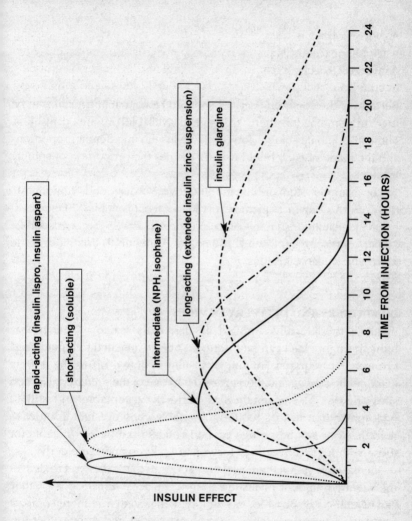

is useful to know where your own brand fits in with the rest if you do have to change for any reason. The main manufacturers are:

- Lilly
- Novo Nordisk
- CP Pharmaceuticals
- Aventis (Hoechst)

Because of the common need for short and longer acting insulins to be used in combination there are several available pre-mixed insulins. These all combine soluble and isophane insulin in different proportions and the name of each brand usually defines the proportion of soluble insulin.

For example, Human Mixtard 30 (Novo Nordisk) and Humulin M3 (Lilly) both contain a mixture of 30 per cent soluble: 70 per cent isophane insulin. Insuman Comb 25 (Aventis) has 25 per cent soluble: 75 per cent isophane insulin, and so on. Appendix B lists most of the presently available insulins.

CONTAINERS AND DELIVERY DEVICES

Insulin is traditionally supplied in glass vials sealed with a rubber bung through which can be inserted a needle attached to a graduated syringe. The required amount of insulin is drawn up to the correct mark on the syringe and then injected into one of the preferred injection sites (figure 7). This method is perfectly acceptable and still in widespread use. It does require reasonably good eyesight in order to read the scale on the syringe properly and so can be less suitable for those with impaired sight or for young children and the elderly.

Increasingly popular are pen-sized devices that can be set to deliver the required amount of insulin from a replaceable cartridge or they can be entirely disposable once empty. Pen systems are more compact and self-contained compared to separate bottles and syringes but it is a good idea for someone with Type 1 to have available vials and syringes as a back-up if their pen system fails and they don't have a readily available spare. The long-acting insulins are in any case only available in vials.

Portable electrically driven pumps are now available that can provide continuous injections of insulin. These can be effective in experienced hands and are most suited to young people with Type 1 diabetes. They are not yet widespread and for many people are less suitable than standard methods using multiple daily injections. In development are inhalers (a bit like those used in asthma) that may be able to deliver insulin via the lungs.

Insulin 'regimes'

By this is meant the pattern in which insulin is used on a regular basis. Whatever regime is chosen it has to do four things well:

1 Provide some insulin continuously for the body's needs
2 Provide boosts of insulin to cope with meals
3 Avoid hypoglycaemic attacks
4 Avoid excessively high peaks of blood glucose

Leaving aside the continuous pump devices, there are three common insulin regimes:

1 Twice daily doses of soluble and isophane insulins
These are given before breakfast and before the evening meal. The soluble doses cover the insulin needs of the morning and evening and the isophane doses cover the afternoon and overnight. The pre-mixed soluble and isophane insulins are convenient for this type of dosing.

2 Three times daily injections
Soluble and isophane before breakfast, soluble before the evening meal and isophane before bed. Moving the second isophane dosage to before bedtime gives better coverage of the overnight period.

3 Multiple daily injections

Soluble insulin is used before each main meal and an intermediate or long-acting insulin is used before bedtime to give coverage overnight.

These three are the commonest regimes but there are others. For example some older individuals can be adequately controlled with a single daily injection of long-acting insulin.

Multiple injections are increasingly being favoured, especially by young people with diabetes, as they give the most flexibility and are the most capable of mimicking natural insulin release. Unfortunately the harder someone tries to keep their blood glucose low the greater is the risk of hypoglycaemic attacks and a balance has always to be struck between the strictness of the glucose control and the need to avoid hypos. It is also important not to turn glucose control into an obsession with over-frequent blood glucose checks and endless fiddling with the insulin dosages.

Hypoglycaemia is a very important aspect of diabetes and is covered in chapter 9.

Keeping a record of blood glucose levels over days and weeks allows one to see the patterns in glucose throughout the day and between different days. This makes it possible to see where changes in insulin dosage or timing are needed, but even so it can take a bit of experience to know how to adjust insulin dosages properly. The diabetic team (GP, nurse, hospital clinic) are there to advise on this aspect of treatment, and will always be willing to do so. Generally speaking small changes to insulin dosage followed by a wait and see policy over at least a few days are much better than trying to make big adjustments that cause erratic glucose changes.

Targets for diabetic control

Human beings are all different, and the aims of treating diabetes are not the same in everyone. In a young to middle aged person with a long life expectancy good diabetic control will reduce the risk of developing long-term complications, and to achieve that will require fairly intensive monitoring and adjustment of the diabetes as required. In an elderly person or someone with a limited outlook for other medical reasons it may be inappropriate to be so precise with the diabetic treatment. Just to control the symptoms of diabetes by reducing excessive blood glucose levels may be all that is required. In this chapter we are dealing with Type 1 diabetes, which usually affects younger people so one is usually attempting to get good control, however the issue of 'how hard to treat' can arise with any of the types of diabetes.

Good control in Type 1 diabetes would be blood glucose consistently between 4 and 7 mmol/l. In turn this should result in an HbA$_{1c}$ of 7 per cent or less. Less strict control, say in which the blood glucose is around 10 mmol/l may be good enough to control symptoms such as thirst and the frequent desire to pass urine and will be acceptable treatment for some people.

Exercise

We've previously mentioned that exercise is an essential part of diabetes treatment. Exercise increases the body's sensitivity to insulin, helps with weight control, encourages the burning of fat and increases muscle mass, all of which improve diabetic control and of course exercise has many other benefits too.

Several quite complex processes normally go on when you undertake exercise so that glucose is made available for the muscles and some understanding of these is essential for a diabetic person. Of particular importance is the effect of a hormone that we've not yet mentioned – adrenaline.

Adrenaline

Adrenaline is a hormone produced by the adrenal glands, which are two walnut-sized pieces of highly specialised tissue that sit on top of each kidney. The adrenal glands are connected by many nerves to the rest of the nervous system and by a rich blood supply to the circulation of the body. They have many important functions, and the release of adrenaline is only one of them. Adrenaline has a powerful effect upon the liver and encourages it to release glucose from its stores of glycogen, thus raising the blood glucose level. One of the effects of vigorous exercise is to stimulate the release of adrenaline from the adrenal glands.

One can see the logic of this – when presented with the need to move in a hurry adrenaline makes glucose readily available for the muscles. However, adrenaline also *reduces* the release of insulin from the pancreas gland. So the effect of adrenaline during exercise is to *increase* the blood glucose.

During exercise the muscles will of course take up glucose from the blood to use as fuel, and this action will *lower* blood glucose. There is therefore a balancing act going on during exercise between the forces that raise and lower glucose.

In a non-diabetic person the body is able to fine tune the release of insulin and adrenaline so that the blood glucose remains pretty constant, but the diabetic person needs to make these adjustments himself. Three factors are at play here – the amount of insulin available, the amount of glucose (food) available and the level of exercise.

Exercise can therefore result in three outcomes for the blood glucose:

1 Too low
This would be caused if there was too much insulin or not enough circulating glucose (or both). This could occur if for example someone was exercising too long after their last meal or if they had taken too much insulin at their last dose. Another cause is injecting the insulin into a limb and then using the limb during exercise. Exercise increases the blood flow to the limbs, which increases the rate at which the insulin is absorbed. It is therefore better to inject insulin into the tummy area if you are then going to go for a run.

2 Too high
The causes could be insufficient insulin available (too little injected at the last dose), or a strong release of glucose from the liver caused by adrenaline, or a big meal shortly before exercising.

3 Normal range

When the correct balance has been struck between the amount of exercise, the dose and timing of insulin and the amount and timing of the last meal.

All of this might make exercise and diabetes look very complicated, which is not the intention. Having diabetes does, however, mean that more thought and planning is required concerning physical activities. Blood glucose testing is essential for someone with Type 1 diabetes who undertakes vigorous exercise so that they get the feel for how their glucose level behaves and then can more accurately judge their insulin and calorie needs.

If, for example, someone takes their normal amount of insulin and a normal meal but then undertakes an unusually large amount of exercise their muscles will use up glucose and a hypo might result. Planning ahead for that exercise, either by taking more food in advance or by reducing the previous insulin dosage slightly would be likely to prevent the hypo from occurring. As muscles continue to 're-fuel' for some hours following vigorous exercise it's also important to realise that the hypo can occur some time later. Carrying extra fluids and glucose supplements is therefore essential for any diabetic person undertaking vigorous exercise or sports.

Gentle exercise is less demanding and needs less planning, although never no planning at all. Once you understand how your own diabetes behaves under different circumstances it will become much easier to keep the glucose levels satisfactory.

Ketones

Ketones are the by-products of the use of fat for energy production and normally only small amounts are produced by the body. In a non-diabetic person ketones will be produced following a period of starvation – they can be detected in the urine by a dipstick test and often can be smelled on the breath of someone who is 'ketotic' as they have a characteristic odour like acetone (nail varnish remover).

In a diabetic person the appearance of ketones usually indicates there is insufficient insulin available and ketones are therefore a sign of poor or impaired diabetic control. This might occur, for example, if the person has an infection, as this is a common reason for the body to temporarily require more insulin. Such illness is often also associated with a drop in appetite, leading to further problems with blood glucose control. It can therefore be useful for a diabetic person to check whether they have ketones with a urine test and to ask their doctor for advice if they appear. Vomiting is particularly likely to cause difficulty with the control of Type 1 diabetes and may in fact be a sign of ketosis, so should always be reported to a doctor.

Key Points

- Type 1 diabetes always needs to be treated with insulin injections.
- The different insulins available vary mainly in the speed with which they are absorbed from the injection site.
- Quick-acting (soluble) insulins are clear.
- Longer-acting insulins are cloudy.
- Insulin regimes vary from once daily to four or more times daily and should be chosen to suit the individual.
- The aim of diabetic treatment is generally to keep blood glucose levels within the 4–7 mmol/l range but for many older people less strict control is adequate.
- Strict glucose control in Type 1 diabetes may be accompanied by increased risk of hypoglycaemic attacks.

Chapter 8

Treatment of Type 2 Diabetes

Not many years ago Type 2 diabetes was commonly thought of as a 'mild' disease, because the symptoms were often controlled with diet, plus or minus tablet treatment. We now know for certain that such a complacent view of Type 2 diabetes is quite wrong. The UKPDS study showed that the better controlled patients with Type 2 diabetes had significantly fewer complications from their diabetes such as eye and kidney disease and were less likely to develop associated problems in the heart and circulation, such as heart attack or stroke. In many ways one has to consider Type 2 diabetes to be as much a disease of the cardiovascular system as it is one of glucose control. This aspect of treatment is covered in more detail in chapter 10.

As with Type 1 diabetes, the aim of treatment is to get the blood glucose level low enough so that the HbA_{1c} is less than 7 per cent. When for various reasons a less strict target is appropriate then an HbA_{1c} of 8 per cent or less should be the goal.

Diet and exercise

As covered in chapter 6, these are always the mainstay of diabetic treatment, but only 20 per cent of people with Type 2 diabetes have their blood glucose levels adequately controlled after 3–12 months on a diet and fewer than 10 per cent are adequately controlled long-term in this way. Diet and exercise are essential though to minimise the need for drug therapy and improve the other aspects of health in diabetes.

Action of drugs in Type 2 diabetes

There are four ways in which drug therapy for Type 2 diabetes can work:

- Reduction of insulin resistance
- Increase in insulin output by the pancreas
- Reduction of the rate of digestion and absorption of carbohydrates from the digestive system
- Insulin treatment

We've already covered insulin treatments in the previous chapter, and in principle the use of insulin in Type 2 follows the same rules. Often the amount of insulin required by a person with Type 2 diabetes of this severity is quite high, as insulin resistance doesn't go away. Leaving aside insulin treatment therefore, we can look at the other three methods of treatment.

DRUGS THAT REDUCE INSULIN RESISTANCE

Insulin resistance is central to Type 2 diabetes so it is logical to use drugs that reduce this effect. There are two sub-groups of drugs in this class (fuller details of the drugs used in treating diabetes are in appendix B).

Biguanide

Metformin is the only drug now available in this group. Metformin increases the sensitivity of tissues to insulin and it also reduces the output of glucose by the liver. It is suitable for overweight people, as it does not have a tendency to promote weight gain. When used on its own it does not cause low blood glucose (hypo) attacks. Metformin therefore tends to be the first choice when an overweight person with Type 2 fails to respond to diet alone. Digestive system upset (diarrhoea) is the main side effect of metformin, although it is usually temporary.

Thiazolidinediones

These new drugs are licensed in the UK for use alongside metformin or with the other drugs that stimulate insulin release (see below). There are two presently in use: pioglitazone and rosiglitazone. Thiazoli-dinediones have other beneficial effects: upon the fat levels in the blood, upon blood pressure and upon the blood's clotting tendency. Their main side effects include weight gain and swelling of the legs (oedema).

DRUGS THAT INCREASE THE RELEASE OF INSULIN FROM THE PANCREAS

Sulphonylureas

These drugs were discovered by chance during research for antibiotics to treat typhoid. It was found that one of the drugs caused blood glucose to fall. Suphonylureas act upon beta cells and stimulate them to release more insulin, so they do not work in the late stages of Type 2, in which beta cells become unable to release any more insulin. They tend to promote weight gain so are best avoided in overweight individuals. They can be used in combination with drugs from the other main groups.

The original sulphonylureas were chlorpropamide and tolbutamide, but chlorpropamide is long-acting, has a tendency to cause hypos and is not now recommended. More recent examples are glibenclamide (also long-acting), gliclazide, glimepiride, glipizide and gliquidone. Suphonylureas are generally well-tolerated drugs, with the main side effect (other than hypos and weight gain) being minor degrees of digestive upset. Rarely they can cause liver inflammation, allergic reactions and blood abnormalities. Many other drugs can clash with the action of sulphonylureas and although outside the scope of this book this is something that needs to be checked by your doctor before prescribing them.

Meglitinides
These drugs stimulate insulin release shortly after they have been taken by mouth so are taken before a meal. Their effect is also short-lived. There are now two available in the UK: nateglinide (which is licensed for use only with metformin) and repaglinide (which can also be used on its own). These drugs can be useful for people with irregular meal patterns.

DRUGS THAT SLOW CARBOHYDRATE DIGESTION
Most of the carbohydrate that we eat is in the form of large molecules that need to be broken down into simpler sugars before being absorbed. This process is carried out by an enzyme present within the lining of the gut. This enzyme is called alpha-glucosidase and drugs that block its action have the effect of slowing the absorption of carbohydrate. This lowers the peak glucose level that occurs after a meal. Acarbose is available in the UK but there are others.

Combining drugs for Type 2 is not straightforward but a general scheme is shown in figure 9. Here all patients are shown to need diet and exercise treatment. When that is insufficient to control the blood glucose (after 3 months' trial) then most will have metformin treatment, except underweight people, who would be better on a sulphonylurea. When that is insufficient then another drug is added. To a sulphonylurea that could be metformin, acarbose or a thiazolidinedione but to metformin it could be a sulphonylurea or a meglitinide or a thiazolidinedione. If that fails then many experts would move to treating with insulin. It is possible to combine insulin with an oral diabetic medicine.

Other factors

Blood glucose control is only one aspect of treating Type 2 diabetes, although a very important one. Attention also has to be directed to reducing obesity, raised blood pressure, raised cholesterol and triglycerides (fats) as well as looking out for the complications of diabetes in the long term.

Figure 9: Scheme of using drugs for Type 2 diabetes

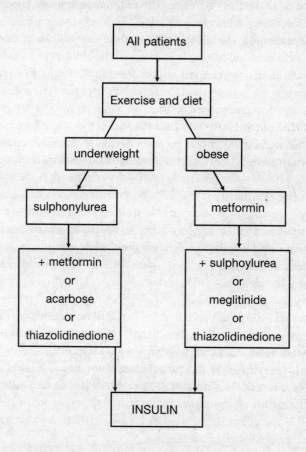

Weight reduction treatment

Many Type 2 patients are too heavy and find it difficult to lose weight. For some it can be helpful to use anti-obesity medication, of which two are presently available in the UK.

Orlistat (Xenical)

This drug reduces the absorption of fat from food by blocking the action of one of the enzymes that digest fat. Its main side effects are flatulence and diarrhoea, which can be minimised by reducing the amount of fat in the diet (which in turn helps weight loss). The National Institute for Clinical Excellence (NICE) has produced guidelines for doctors concerning the appropriate use of orlistat. In diabetes the recommendations include that a person should have a body mass index of 28 or more (chapter 6) before considering the use of the drug. Using it for longer than three or six months is recommended only if there has been weight loss of 5 per cent and 10 per cent respectively from the start. Orlistat only works to reduce fat absorption – it will not reduce weight on its own. Similarly if a meal contains no fat then the relevant dose of orlistat should be omitted.

Sibutramine (Reductil)

This drug is related to modern antidepressants and promotes a feeling of fullness after a meal. It is not suitable for people with a history of heart disease and a number of other conditions and it can cause the blood pressure to rise. As with orlistat, NICE has produced guidelines concerning its use.

Although these drugs do have a place in the management of obesity in general, and particularly when there are other significant health problems such as diabetes present, they are appropriate for only a very small proportion of the population. They are not without their own problems too, so a decision to use them has to be made on the basis of knowing all the facts.

Chapter 9

Hypoglycaemia

Brain and nervous tissues are completely dependent upon circulating glucose for their energy needs and are very sensitive to falls in blood glucose. Once the glucose level drops below 3 mmol/l then 'hypoglycaemia' is technically said to exist and at this level the majority of people will start to have symptoms.

These symptoms reflect both the response of the body to try to correct the low blood glucose and the direct effects upon the nervous system and brain when they have insufficient energy to function properly. The level of glucose required for hypoglycaemic symptoms to arise is not the same in all people. Although most people will get symptoms at or below 3 mmol/l some people will feel 'hypo' at higher levels than this, especially if they have been used to high glucose levels most of the time.

Symptoms from the corrective responses of the body

These are largely the result of the release of adrenaline. Adrenaline has a powerful effect upon the liver and stimulates it to release stored glucose; however, it also causes a rapid pulse, sweating, tremor and a feeling of anxiety.

Symptoms from the nervous system

These include a feeling of hunger, faintness and headache, odd behaviour and confusion, drowsiness and eventually coma.

Importance of hypo attacks

Virtually everyone with Type 1 diabetes and many people with Type 2 will experience some hypo attacks. Many of these attacks are mild and if recognised in time they can be reversed by taking extra glucose right away. If the signs are not recognised and go on long enough to result in diabetic coma then the results can be serious.

If the brain is starved of glucose for a prolonged period of time there is a risk of brain damage. People who are deeply unconscious, for any reason, are exposed to risks from many directions such as inhaling vomit if they are sick. Hypo attacks are therefore to be avoided if at all possible.

Dealing with hypos

The signs of a hypo attack should be known not only by the diabetic person but also by those around them, such as work colleagues and relatives. The initial signs might be quite mild and the pattern can be fairly similar from attack to attack, so recognising the pattern early on will hopefully alert the diabetic person or the observer to act quickly. A conscious person should be encouraged to take a quickly absorbed sugary drink or sweet food. Glucose tablets are ideal. If unconsciousness occurs then it will usually be necessary for a doctor or paramedic to inject concentrated glucose solution through a vein. Glucagon can however be injected easily into a muscle and in many people it will be rapidly effective in raising the blood glucose. An important exception is if the hypo has been brought on by alcohol, which blocks the effect of glucagon.

Although someone with a hypo might be brought round quite quickly with extra glucose they might not be immediately out of trouble. If, for example, the hypo has been caused by an excess of long-acting insulin or especially if it is due to an overdose of a sulphonylurea drug then the person may be at risk of becoming hypoglycaemic again once the boost of glucose wears off.

Hypos due to sulphonylurea drugs should be treated in hospital and in some cases the patient may need to be observed for several days before the risk of hypoglycaemia passes completely.

LACK OF WARNING SIGNS

Some people get little warning of hypos and are therefore at particular risk from them. Hypos are commonest in people with Type 1 diabetes who try to maintain tight blood glucose control, and having frequent hypos tends to reduce people's sensitivity to the early signs of them occurring.

When human insulins first became available in the 1980s some people who were transferred from animal insulin felt they had fewer warning symptoms of hypoglycaemia. This has never been convincingly proved to be true, and it seems more likely that the hypos related more to tighter control of the blood glucose. Some drugs, notably beta-blockers (usually used for angina or high blood pressure) dampen the body's response to hypoglycaemia.

Night-time hypos

Hypos that occur during the night can present several difficulties. As the person is asleep they can be completely unaware that a hypo has occurred, even if quite a low blood glucose has occurred. Very low blood glucose levels are dangerous and so measures need to be taken to avoid night-time hypos as much as possible. There is no single best way of doing this but checking the glucose level before bed, taking a bedtime snack and ensuring that the long-acting insulin dose before bed is not excessive are all important.

It is important to keep hypos in perspective. True, they can be dangerous if severe but very few people with diabetes get away with never having a hypo attack. Most are accompanied by some warning symptoms that should be looked out for and ready access to quick-acting glucose sweets is essential, especially for those people with Type 1 who are trying for good glucose control.

Key Points

- Hypoglycaemia (low blood sugar) is defined as a blood glucose of less than 3 mmol/l.
- Symptoms of hypoglycaemia can occur at higher blood glucose levels than this.
- The possible warning symptoms of a hypo attack should be known by the diabetic person and by those around them.
- First aid treatment of a hypo in a conscious person is to give fast-acting sugary foods or drinks.
- Unconsciousness from diabetic coma is a medical emergency and urgent assistance should always be obtained for it.
- Glucagon injected into a muscle usually works well for a hypo not associated with alcohol.
- Hypos are potentially dangerous and good diabetic treatment aims to minimise their occurrence.

Chapter 10

Diabetes and the Circulation

There are many aspects to the need to detect and deal with diabetes. For the person with recent onset Type 1 diabetes who has developed ketoacidosis the prompt diagnosis and treatment of his condition may be life-saving. The majority of people with diabetes do not develop such an urgent and immediately threatening complication as this. Everyone with diabetes – of all types – is, however, potentially at risk of developing the long-term consequences of the condition. The purpose of treatment is to reduce or eliminate some or all of these complications by careful attention to all aspects of diabetes.

The rest of this chapter will deal with the common factor that runs through all of the long-term problems associated with diabetes – its effect upon the circulation. Following chapters deal with the particular problems associated with eyes, kidneys and the nervous system that are seen in diabetes.

High glucose levels, if present for lengthy periods of months or years, damage the microscopic structure of the smallest arteries of the body. We do not know why this is so. It is important to note that it is the high glucose level that does the damage, so the long-term complications occur in all types of diabetes. The complications become more severe with:

- the length of time diabetes has been present;
- the proportion of the time that blood glucose levels are high.

Consequently the problems of diabetes can be lessened with good treatment that keeps the glucose level in check. Diagnosing diabetes early is, as we've seen, a problem in Type 2 diabetes because the symptoms can be fairly mild and unfortunately many people already have some complications at the time their diabetes is detected.

Small and large vessel disease

The structure of our circulation is very much like the branching of a tree. The single main artery that leaves the heart (aorta) repeatedly divides and sends branches to the main regions of the body. These arteries subdivide time and again until every part of the body has been reached. The smallest blood vessels are the capillaries, which are just a few thousandths of a millimetre across. These vessels, and the tiny arteries that supply them, are collectively called the 'microcirculation'. It is at this level that the characteristic changes of diabetes occur. Doctors usually refer to these as the 'microvascular' or 'small vessel' changes of diabetes. The processes that go on in these very small blood vessels as a result of prolonged high glucose levels are being researched very actively but basically the vessels become more 'leaky' and let through large molecules such as proteins that would not normally be able to get through the lining of the small arteries. There are also abnormalities of blood flow and blood clotting. The end result is poorer delivery of oxygen to the tissues, particularly to the eyes, kidneys and nerves. Shortly we'll discuss each of these in detail.

Diabetes also accelerates the process of hardening and blockage of the arteries that is common in most people as they get older, whether or not they have diabetes. This is called 'atherosclerosis' or 'arteriosclerosis' – they both mean the same thing. Atherosclerosis is also commoner in people who smoke, have high blood pressure and high blood cholesterol levels. Atherosclerosis has many serious effects depending on which parts of the blood vessel system it affects. In the heart arteries it causes angina and heart attacks (coronary heart disease), in the brain it leads to stroke and in the limbs it can cause poor circulation, which sometimes leads to the need for amputation. Because all of these complications are the result of blockage of the larger arteries they are called the 'macrovascular' or 'large vessel' changes of diabetes.

Note that large vessel disease, unlike small vessel disease, is not unique to diabetes. However, the effect diabetes has upon large vessel disease is very marked. Having diabetes:

- doubles a man's risk and quadruples (x four) a woman's risk of having a heart attack;
- doubles the risk of someone having a stroke;
- quadruples the risk of developing severe problems with the circulation to the legs.

Risk factors

These are hard facts, and not pleasant reading if you have diabetes. However the risks can be substantially reduced, not just by making sure that you get your diabetes under good control and keep it that way, but also by vigorously tackling the other 'risk factors' that contribute to anyone developing atherosclerosis. We've covered these points already, but to recap:

- *Smoking.* Smoking is bad news for everyone, but particularly so in diabetes. The number one priority for any diabetic who smokes is to pack it in.

- **High blood pressure.** Good blood pressure control is essential in diabetic people, for whom the targets are more rigorous than the average population.
- **Overweight.** The majority of people with Type 2 diabetes are overweight. Reducing weight can markedly improve the diabetes, and it reduces the risk of atherosclerosis too.
- **High blood fat levels.** Cholesterol and triglyceride are the two main fats that circulate in the blood. Raised cholesterol in particular is associated with atherosclerosis, and again the targets for lowering cholesterol in diabetes are tougher than average.

The above are the 'modifiable' risk factors – the ones you can do something about. The two other main risk factors for atherosclerosis in diabetes are not ones you can change:

- **Age.** Atherosclerosis is commoner in older people.
- **Length of time diabetic.** As far as Type 1 diabetes is concerned we do not have any way of postponing its onset and you have to live with it once it is there. So you can't make much change to the date at which you develop diabetes. Although this is largely true also for Type 2 diabetes there can be exceptions. If someone who might go on to be diabetic and who is overweight and sedentary gets their weight down and becomes more active then diabetes may be staved off – possibly permanently but at least for a worthwhile amount of time. The message is of course that it's better to improve your health 'before you need to' rather than afterwards – you could save yourself a lot of trouble.

Blood pressure

Raised blood pressure is an important issue in diabetes and deserves a bit of explanation. It is covered fully in a companion book in this series, so only the most important facts are presented here.

Each beat of the heart sends a pulse of pressure through all of the arteries of the body, propelling blood around the circulation. The maximum pressure developed during this action is called the 'systolic pressure'. Blood pressure falls while the heart is re-filling in readiness for the next beat, but not to zero – the minimum pressure reached at this part of the cycle is the 'diastolic pressure'. Blood pressure is always measured in millimetres of mercury (written as mmHg), which comes from the fact that blood pressure measuring devices use the height of a column of mercury as the standard against which to gauge the pressure.

In diabetes the top level of acceptable systolic pressure is 140 mmHg (British Hypertension Society guidelines) and of diastolic pressure it is 80 mmHg. The shorthand way of writing this blood pressure is 140/80. Increasingly some experts are advising that a tighter target of 130 mmHg is desirable in diabetes, especially if kidney complications are present (chapter 12). If either of the systolic or diastolic readings is consistently above these levels then treatment to lower the blood pressure to within target levels is required. This might mean simple dietary salt restriction and weight loss if the rise is small, or long-term blood pressure lowering medication if simple measures fail.

If you do have raised blood pressure the most useful things you can do to help yourself are:

- *Reduce the amount of salt in your diet.* Remember you should take less than 5 grams of salt daily, including all of the salt that comes in processed foods.
- *Increase the amount of fresh fruit and vegetables in your diet.* These contain potassium, which is also a salt but unlike sodium, which is common table salt and bad for blood pressure, increased potassium in the diet helps lower blood pressure.
- *Take more exercise.* You don't need to become an athlete to get the benefits. A brisk walk three times a week lasting about 20–40 minutes will lower blood pressure.
- *Keep alcohol consumption to about one or two units daily.* Consuming a small amount of alcohol daily (up to two standard units) appears to have a beneficial effect upon cardiovascular risk. There are many possible explanations for this, but among the most

likely are that compounds within some alcoholic drinks, particularly red wine, mop up 'free radical' molecules that are capable of causing tissue damage. However the effects rapidly turn from beneficial to harmful when higher levels of alcohol are consumed.

- ***Keep your body weight to the ideal range.*** This will also make it much easier to achieve good blood glucose control.

All of the above are standard things that anyone with high blood pressure can do to help themselves. The only difference for a diabetic person is that the dietary recommendations need to be taken into account within their daily calorie allowance.

Key Points

- Small vessel changes are unique to diabetes and particularly affect the eyes, kidneys and nerves.
- Large vessel changes can affect anyone but are more pronounced in diabetes.
- Improvement in modifiable risk factors lessens the development of all forms of blood vessel disease in diabetes, and their consequences.
- In diabetes the blood pressure should be kept to 140/80 mmHg or below.

Chapter 11

Diabetes and the Eye

Losing one's sight is one of the most dreaded complications any disease could have and in young to middle aged people, diabetes is the commonest cause of blindness. Fortunately such an outcome affects only a minority of diabetic people. Lesser degrees of diabetic eye disease are however common and can give rise to significant visual problems. At any one point in time about 10 per cent of diabetic people have eye disease that requires treatment and/or monitoring by an eye specialist. Up to 90 per cent of people who have had diabetes for 20 years will show some effects upon the eyes.

Diabetic eye disease generally is a slow enough process to allow it to be detected and acted upon in people who are known to have diabetes and who attend a regular and effective screening programme. You will be well aware by now though that many people with Type 2 diabetes go undetected for months or years. By the time that they are diagnosed 39 per cent have diabetic eye disease, with 4–8 per cent having sight-threatening levels of eye involvement. Some of those who *are* diagnosed don't attend for screening, so they miss the benefit of having their eyes checked properly and for corrective action to be taken if changes are beginning to appear. Screening programmes themselves are generally well organised in the UK – there is no excuse for a known diabetic person to receive other than excellent eye care, provided they attend for their checks. Although only the earliest phases of eye damage can be reversed with treatment the progress of more advanced damage can usually be markedly slowed down, avoiding serious threat to sight.

Diabetes affects both the front and the back of the eye. At the front is the lens, clouding of which is called cataract – a common finding in all older people and in fact the commonest cause of visual impairment in people with Type 2 diabetes, who are of course usually older than those with Type 1. Type 2, however, doubles the chance of developing cataract.

The light sensitive part of the eye, at the back, is the retina and the medical term for the eye damage that occurs here is 'retinopathy'. This is where the most serious and specific diabetic eye trouble is located.

Inspecting the eyes

The retina can be inspected by a doctor or optician using the hand-held illuminated magnifier called an ophthalmoscope, which is a common piece of medical equipment. High quality cameras are now routinely used to take photographs of the retina both in eye clinics and increasingly in well-equipped high street opticians. Photographs allow detailed examination of the retina at leisure and provide a permanent record that tracks the progress of retinopathy and its treatment.

A 'slit lamp' is a type of microscope that gives a good view of the eye. Both the patient and the examiner sit down on either side of this instrument, the patient with his or her chin on a rest, and the examiner can then move the microscope and light source around to get a good view. Slit lamp microscopes are expensive and are not part of the equipment used by GPs. Your optician should however have access to one, and it is standard equipment in a hospital eye clinic.

Stages of retinopathy

There are several recognised stages in diabetic retinopathy. First the small vessels swell slightly and then they develop small blebs, called 'microaneurysms' on their surface. These blebs show up as tiny red dots scattered on the retina. They are leaky and allow through proteins from the blood, which settle around the vessels, forming whitish spots called 'hard exudates'. Blood can also leak out from weakened vessels, causing small collections of blood (haemorrhages) to appear.

Changes to this stage (microaneurysms, hard exudates and haemorrhages) are called 'background' or 'simple' retinopathy – although neither term is meant to imply that such changes are unimportant, because they certainly are. Whether this stage of retinopathy affects a person's eyesight depends entirely on which part of the retina is affected. Although all of the retina is sensitive to light there is a small part that we use much more than the rest and which is very important in seeing small details. It's a region called the macula, and light from straight in front of the eye naturally falls upon this part of the retina (see figure 10). If haemorrhages or exudates are deposited here then eyesight can be affected but if the macula is free of such changes then there may not be much visual loss at this stage.

In the next stages of retinopathy some of the small vessels close, thus cutting down the supply of blood (and hence oxygen) to the parts of the retina they serve. These retinal areas look pale and have indistinct edges, hence their name of 'cotton wool spots'. What happens now is a response of the eye to the lack of blood getting through to various parts of the retina – new blood vessels sprout from the adjacent arteries and start to migrate in towards the affected areas. These new vessels are, however, fragile, prone to leaking and haemorrhaging and they also get stuck to the 'jelly' of the eye. These 'adhesions' contract and can lift off the retina from its base. All of these processes disrupt the function of the retina and can seriously impair vision. If a large

Figure 10: Section through the right eye, seen from above

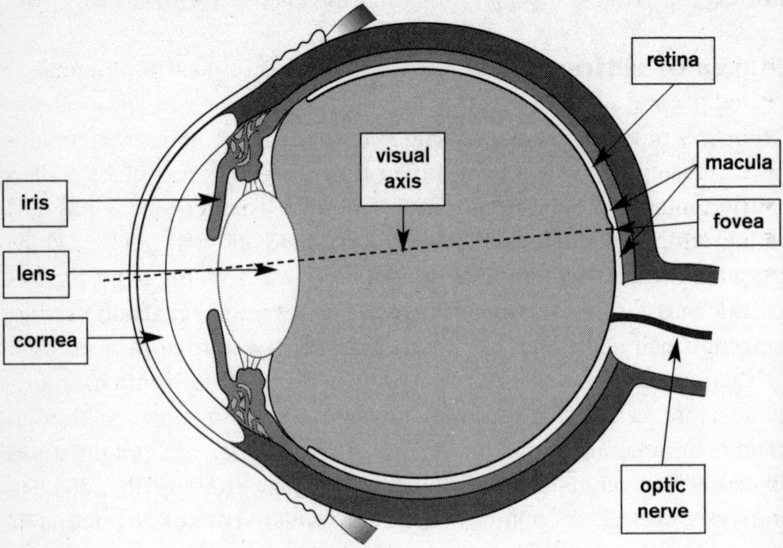

haemorrhage occurs it can also block out a major part of the retina, and in the process permanently damage the blood supply to the retina.

This more advanced stage is called 'proliferative retinopathy', referring to the new vessel formation that goes on and 'pre-proliferative', which is the stage just before new vessels start appearing. Proliferative retinopathy occurs in about 10 per cent of people with diabetes (especially those with long-standing Type 1) and it is a serious threat to sight. Without treatment half of such people will be blind in five years.

Prevention and treatment of retinopathy

As with all diabetic complications, they are lessened when the diabetes is well controlled. It is essential to detect Type 2 diabetes at the earliest stage, which implies that we have got to start looking for it in apparently healthy individuals.

The risk factors that increase the rate at which retinopathy occurs include:

- poor blood glucose control, i.e. too high, too much of the time;
- high blood pressure;
- length of time diabetes has been present;
- increasing number of microaneurysms;
- presence of protein in the urine (see next chapter);
- raised triglycerides (fats) in the blood;
- pregnancy. (This happens to a small number of pregnant women but only those who already have diabetes and background retinopathy before becoming pregnant. Retinopathy does not occur in pure 'pregnancy diabetes'.)

There is some debate about whether smoking makes retinopathy more likely and the consensus view is that it probably does in Type 1. The need for diabetic people to be non-smokers has already been mentioned. The two most important risk factors that one should improve to reduce the chances of getting retinopathy are glucose control and blood pressure.

Screening for eye disease

Detection and monitoring of retinopathy requires a combined approach between the patient, GP practice, regional diabetes service, eye specialist and possibly opticians. All adults with diabetes should be screened annually with ophthalmoscopy, retinal photographs or a slit lamp microscope.

If someone with diabetes has no retinopathy at diagnosis the chance of him or her developing it within the next two years is low – less than 1 per cent. If there is any retinopathy that could possibly affect vision then an eye specialist (ophthalmologist) should see the patient. The frequency of screening may need to be increased if there is more significant retinopathy, or to monitor treatment.

Treatment

The main treatment method is multiple pulses of laser light applied across the retina and also directed at 'leaky' vessels to seal them. Laser treatment reduces the tendency for more new vessels to form but it can only preserve sight, not retrieve lost sight. The results of treatment depend a bit on which part of the retina is involved – results are less good for the macula.

Surgical treatment to remove cataract is just as successful in diabetes but may need to be done at an earlier stage than in non-diabetics to allow a good enough view of the retina if retinopathy is present and needs monitoring or treatment.

It is possible to remove the 'jelly' (vitreous) from within the eyeball if it is scarred or distorting the retina or if there has been bleeding behind it which is not clearing away with time. This operation is called 'vitrectomy'.

Key Points

- Diabetic eye disease affects both Type 1 and Type 2 diabetes.
- Retinopathy is the process of blockage followed by leakage of the very small blood vessels that travel across the surface of the retina.
- Retinopathy can be slowed down by good glucose control and by minimising other risk factors, particularly high blood pressure.

- Eye screening should be at least annually in diabetes and by ophthalmoscopy, retinal photographs and/or slit lamp examination.
- Laser treatment can be used in diabetic eye disease and it slows or prevents the deterioration of eyesight that can occur in untreated patients.

- **Any sudden loss or change in vision should be treated as a medical emergency (whether or not diabetes is present) and requires prompt medical assessment.**

Chapter 12

Diabetes and the Kidney

Through the changes in small vessels explained in chapter 5, diabetes can damage the kidneys and in a significant proportion of people severe kidney failure can eventually result. Subtle kidney involvement can be shown to start within a year or so of Type 1 diabetes and can be present at diagnosis in Type 2 diabetes but it usually takes 5–10 years to become a noticeable problem. The medical term for the kidney disease seen in diabetes is 'nephropathy'.

There are wide differences in estimates of how many people with diabetes will progress to having nephropathy. 6–27 per cent of people with Type 1 and 25–50 per cent of Type 2 may do so. Factors that increase the risk of making kidney disease worse follow a pattern that will now be familiar to you – poor glucose control is one of the main ones and even modestly high blood pressure can significantly accelerate the condition. Racial origin is very important in Type 2 diabetes – people from an Asian or

Afro-Caribbean origin are twice as likely to develop nephropathy as Europeans.

Significance of nephropathy

The kidneys are essential organs. They filter and eliminate the waste products of metabolism, have a central role in controlling blood pressure and fluid balance in the body and produce the key hormone that stimulates the bone marrow to manufacture red blood cells – to name a few of their roles. Although we have quite a bit of spare capacity in the kidney system the loss of kidney function from any cause is a potentially serious matter. Diabetic nephropathy is the commonest cause of advanced renal failure. People with very poor kidney function require some form of artificial kidney support (dialysis) or a kidney transplant. The increasing numbers of people with Type 2 diabetes especially has meant that the demand for these facilities has been steadily climbing for several years.

Because the kidneys have a very important role in the control of blood pressure it is common for people with nephropathy to have raised blood pressure. High blood pressure accelerates the decline in kidney function in nephropathy – in other words the two problems multiply each other's effect. By lowering the blood pressure to quite strict levels nephropathy can be slowed down.

Protein in the urine

The marker that shows nephropathy has appeared is the presence of protein in the urine. Proteins are large molecules and are normally kept almost completely out of the urine because of the effectiveness of the kidney filtering system. In nephropathy, however, the filters become leaky and start to let protein through. Albumin is a natural protein that is detected by urine tests for nephropathy. Modern test techniques can detect much lower amounts of albumin than used to be possible, hence the term 'microalbuminuria' has arisen. This means an amount of albumin in the urine of between 30 and 300 milligrams (mg) per day. Smaller amounts than this are normal. When the amount detected goes over 300mg per day then nephropathy is deemed to have started in earnest. Doctors usually use the word 'proteinuria' to mean that there is protein in the urine to this extent or greater.

Microalbuminuria is not a harmless stage that can be ignored until proteinuria starts. People with microalbuminuria are two to four times more likely to develop heart disease (coronary artery disease) than the average person of the same age.

- Microalbuminuria indicates that some kidney disease (nephropathy) is present.
- Proteinuria signals a more advanced stage of nephropathy in which worsening kidney function and other complications such as coronary heart disease develop more rapidly.

There are other possible causes of protein appearing in the urine, of which the commonest is a urine infection. This is tested by sending a sample of urine to the laboratory, where it will be examined for the presence of bacteria. It is always important to check for infection when protein is first found in the urine.

SCREENING
Checking the urine for albumin is therefore an important part of diabetes management and should be done at least annually. A sample from the first urine passed in the morning can be used as a quick check and if it shows a very low concentration of albumin then all is well for the present. If the concentration is higher then slightly more sophisticated tests are done on a longer collection of urine to accurately measure the amount being passed. Test kits are now available that allow quick checks to be done in your GP's surgery but all GPs have access to laboratory testing for the accurate measurement of protein in the urine.

Checking kidney function

Checking for protein in the urine is one way of detecting kidney damage but blood tests are how the overall efficiency of the kidneys is measured. Urea and creatinine are natural compounds present in the blood that are formed by the normal metabolism of protein such as muscles in the body. It is one of the jobs of the kidney to eliminate excess urea and creatinine through the urine, and levels of these two substances start to climb if kidney function becomes poorer.

Risk factors for nephropathy

This list has some things in common with that for retinopathy, and some differences. The main ones are:

- poor blood glucose control i.e. too high, too much of the time;
- high blood pressure;
- length of time diabetes has been present;
- presence of retinopathy;
- degree of protein in the urine;
- raised cholesterol and triglycerides (fats) in the blood;
- age (increased risk with increasing age);
- smoking (definitely this time);
- male sex.

Acting on protein in the urine

You could say that detecting microalbuminuria should not really make any difference to the need to control diabetes and all the associated risk factors because they should always be treated as well as possible. In an ideal world that would be true, but treatment is rarely at its best in anyone. However the appearance of microalbuminuria means that extra effort needs to be applied to improve the treatment. The diabetic person can help themselves enormously by giving up smoking and complying as much as possible with their diabetic treatment so that blood glucose levels are as good as possible. The doctor can help by ensuring that blood pressure control is rigorously kept below 140/80 mmHg and, preferably, should be 130/80 or less. The benefit of putting off or avoiding further falls in kidney function with all that goes with it are well worth striving for.

ACE inhibitor drugs

This is a group of drugs invented primarily as treatment for high blood pressure but which have been shown to significantly reduce the loss of albumin through the kidneys in diabetic nephropathy. ACE inhibitors are very effective drugs for lowering blood pressure but they also appear to have extra benefits on the heart and kidneys on top of their blood pressure lowering ability. For example they reduce the likelihood of heart attack in Type 2 diabetes by 25 per cent when given over several years and in Type 1 patients with nephropathy who were given these drugs over three years a 50 per cent reduction was seen in all events including dialysis, kidney transplantation and death.

Angiotensin converting enzyme (ACE) is present in lung tissue and is one of the many components of the body's inbuilt mechanisms for controlling blood pressure. Blockage of this enzyme with the ACE inhibitor drugs lowers blood pressure. ACE inhibitors are well-tolerated drugs that can be given to a wide range of people. The most common side effect is a dry cough that can be troublesome enough to make the drug intolerable. It is caused by the action of ACE inhibitors on another enzyme within the lung. Very rarely a severe allergic reaction develops to ACE inhibitors.

The ACE inhibitors commonly in use are: captopril, lisinopril, ramipril, cilazapril, enalapril, fosinopril, imidapril, moexipril, perindopril, quinapril, and trandolapril.

Angiotensin II receptor blockers

These drugs block a different chemical step in blood pressure control within the body although the end result is similar to the ACE inhibitors in the way they work. Their main advantage is their remarkably low tendency to cause side effects – in particular they do not cause cough. As yet they have not been shown to be superior to ACE inhibitors in treating high blood pressure, which is their main area of application, but large studies investigating their role are under way.

Like ACE inhibitors, angiotensin II receptor blockers have also been shown to be beneficial in diabetic nephropathy. In one study the number of people with Type 2 diabetes and microalbuminuria who went on to develop proteinuria over two years was reduced by two thirds, independently of their blood pressure level. The angiotensin II blockers presently in use in the UK are losartan, valsartan, candesartan, eprosartan, irbesartan and telmisartan.

Although ACE inhibitors and angiotensin II receptor blockers can be given to a wide range of people, they are not suitable for everyone. People with widespread atherosclerosis may have reduced blood supply to the kidneys and they can develop a worsening of kidney function on these drugs. Judgement is therefore required when prescribing them and blood checks on kidney function need to be done shortly after starting them to ensure that they are not causing problems.

Most diabetic people with proteinuria should be started on an ACE inhibitor or an angiotensin II receptor blocker, provided there are no other conditions barring their use.

When kidney function gets worse

Despite everyone's best efforts it may be impossible to prevent the kidneys from slowly deteriorating. As they do so then the blood levels of urea and creatinine begin to climb, and many other problems also occur within the fluid and salt balance of the body, which the healthy kidney takes care of automatically.

Initially dietary restriction of protein and fluid intake will reduce the workload of the kidney and can slow the rate of any deterioration. When that fails to work then other techniques to help or replace the kidney function are needed.

Dialysis is the term for these techniques. One method is the 'artificial kidney' – a sophisticated filter that removes excess waste compounds from the patient's blood. These machines work well but they usually need to be sited in a dialysis unit, which involves travelling to and from the unit two, three or four times a week, each session lasting several hours.

Over the last 20 or so years a simpler but much more convenient type of dialysis has been developed which can be carried out at home and requires very little equipment. This is called 'continuous ambulatory peritoneal dialysis', or CAPD for short.

CAPD takes advantage of the fact that inside the abdomen the membrane that covers all of the organs, called the peritoneum, is a semi-permeable membrane. In CAPD a flexible, perforated plastic tube is introduced through the skin of the abdomen and anchored there. This tube is of a non-irritating material and it can be left in place for several weeks before it needs to be replaced. Inside the abdomen the tube lies within the folds of the peritoneum, but outside the digestive system. The outer part of the tube can be connected to bags of specially designed fluid which are made up to contain the correct balance of salts that the body should have. These bags are made to be free of any bacteria and careful technique on the part of the patient is necessary to prevent any infection when connecting and disconnecting the bags.

To carry out a dialysis a bag of fluid is run into the abdomen, left for a few hours and then run out again and discarded. During the time that the fluid is inside the abdomen an exchange of salts and fluid takes place across the peritoneum, which results in a cleaning effect of the person's blood. CAPD can be carried out repeatedly and may be the only type of dialysis someone needs.

With good care of diabetes and associated factors such as high blood pressure only a small proportion of people who have diabetes will need to consider this type of treatment. The increasing total numbers of diabetic people are however tending to push up the number of people who develop severe kidney problems. Dialysis is a successful technique that can be done well and allows most people to feel very much better.

Kidney transplantation is the only way for someone with severe kidney failure to receive long-term treatment that does not depend on machines or other equipment, and diabetic people can receive a kidney transplant as successfully as any other person.

Chapter 13

Diabetes and the Nervous System

Another of the 'small vessel disease' complications of diabetes is impairment of function of nerve fibres. The commonest form this takes is damage to the nerves that serve sensation in the feet. Usually each foot is equally affected and as time goes on the problem spreads up the legs. As a consequence there may be poor sensation in the feet, making them more prone to injury. Combined with poor circulation this can easily lead to ulcers and infection in the feet, which is one of the important things that good diabetic care tries to avoid.

The sensory nervous system

The commonest type of damage to nerves seen in diabetes is that of impaired sensation. An early sign of it is a lack of ability to feel vibrations, for example from a tuning fork – a common test that can be used by a doctor in a diabetic check-up. The same sort of nerve damage can occur in the hands but it is uncommon, and is always accompanied by problems in the feet and legs. Unfortunately this type of nerve damage is permanent and, once it has occurred, it is not improved by better diabetic control. Good control does however reduce the chance of it occurring in the first place.

Other types of nerve damage seen in diabetes include paralysis involving single nerves and some painful types of neuralgia. These particular nerve conditions can be improved by good diabetic control after they have occurred.

The 'autonomic' nervous system

This is the part of the nervous system that works in the background, so to speak, controlling our blood pressure, temperature, breathing, pulse rate, digestive system and so on. The fibres of the autonomic system reach every part of the body and ultimately are connected to the brain and spinal cord.

Damage to these nerve fibres is another consequence of long-standing diabetes and has many potential consequences depending on which body system is involved. The main ones are:

1 Digestive system
Diarrhoea, which is usually intermittent and can be controlled with medicines to slow the bowels.

2 Blood pressure control
Loss of the normal reflexes that increase our blood pressure when we stand up. As a result this can cause marked dizziness on standing, sometimes enough to cause the person to faint.

3 Erectile dysfunction (impotence)
The process of erection of the penis in a man is a complex one and involves many steps, from the brain, through the spinal cord and nerves to the penis as well as its blood supply, all of which can be badly affected in diabetes. As many as a third of men with diabetes experience

erectile dysfunction. Treatment used to be fairly disappointing but sildenafil (Viagra) has made a substantial difference and now over 70 per cent of men can be treated successfully. Those with very poor circulation may, however, not respond very well. Two other drugs like sildenafil are due to be released later in 2002. Men who have erectile dysfunction secondary to diabetes are entitled to have sildenafil prescribed under the National Health Service. Other treatments for erectile dysfunction include injections or implants of drugs to stimulate an erection and other physical aids including, very occasionally, surgical implants.

Diabetic foot care

As a consequence of impaired sensation minor injuries to the feet (and sometimes quite major ones) can go unnoticed. Added to the sensation problem is the increased chance of a diabetic person having poor circulation, so foot care is especially important in diabetes. As well as self-awareness and regular checking, annual feet inspections should be a routine part of the care provided by the diabetic team and access to a chiropodist should be readily available for those who need it. Well-fitting shoes are a must and when poor sensation does exist special care should be taken to avoid injury, including when cutting toenails. Any cuts, blisters or infections should be checked by the diabetes nurse or doctor if they are at all slow to heal.

Chapter 14

Diabetes and Pregnancy

Diabetes, particularly if poorly controlled, can reduce fertility slightly but a diabetic woman is unlikely to have particular problems conceiving. Looking at the problem the other way round, a fairly common condition called polycystic ovary syndrome (PCOS), which is associated with infertility, is also associated with the development of Type 2 diabetes. Pregnancy can potentially have significant effects upon diabetes, and vice versa, so it is very important that a diabetic woman who intends to become pregnant discusses the implications for herself and the child well in advance with her GP and other members of the diabetic team. In addition to those who have pre-existing diabetes a group of women develop diabetes during the pregnancy. This is called gestational diabetes and it also requires special consideration.

Pre-existing diabetes

The majority of diabetic women who become pregnant have Type 1 diabetes but increasing numbers of women with Type 2 diabetes are being seen. As with all types of diabetes, good blood glucose control is the key aim before, during and after pregnancy. Babies born to mothers with poor blood glucose control are more likely to have birth defects or to be stillborn. The weight of babies born to diabetic mothers is greater than average, especially if the glucose control is poor during the pregnancy.

For the mother, diabetes and pregnancy can be associated with extra risks. Retinopathy may sometimes increase in severity quite markedly and this is more likely if the mother also has diabetic kidney disease. Diabetic nephropathy increases the chance of her developing high blood pressure or the more serious condition called pre-eclampsia in which high blood pressure is associated with further kidney changes. These conditions are associated with increased risk to the baby too.

Establishing good glucose control well in advance of the pregnancy (so-called 'pre-pregnancy care') and maintaining that control reduces the chance of all these problems occurring. A combined approach between the woman and her GP, nurses, eye specialist (when necessary) and the obstetrician is the best way to minimise problems.

Type 2 oral hypoglycaemic drugs are not recommended in pregnancy and so women with Type 2 diabetes are advised to convert to insulin treatment before becoming pregnant.

Regular blood glucose checks are essential to keep track of the diabetes as the increasing demands of the growing baby combined with the natural tendency for insulin resistance to increase in all pregnancies mean that the mother's insulin requirement will increase as the pregnancy develops.

Full term in pregnancy is 40 weeks but many labours in diabetic mothers are induced (started early) at 38 to 39 weeks to reduce the risk of stillbirth. As a result Caesarian section deliveries are commoner in diabetic mothers. From the start of the second trimester of pregnancy (13 weeks onwards) blood pressure and glucose levels can start to increase more rapidly, so need more frequent monitoring. Once labour starts then insulin and glucose are given by drip feeds, adjusted to keep the blood sugar level. Most babies born to diabetic mothers are healthy and do not routinely require special care but special attention is taken to ensure the baby is not hypoglycaemic at birth.

Gestational diabetes

Resistance to insulin develops in all mothers during pregnancy and in about 2–4 per cent of women this will result in a temporary diabetic state. This is because these women have less ability to produce extra insulin to overcome the insulin resistance. Half of women who have gestational diabetes go on to develop Type 2 diabetes within 10–15 years of giving birth.

Gestational diabetes is more likely in older women (over 25) who are overweight, smoke, have a family history of diabetes and are from an ethnic minority group. Routine antenatal checks include checking the urine for glucose but this is unreliable as a test for any form of diabetes and all women should at least have a fasting or random blood glucose checked between 26 and 30 weeks of pregnancy. Women who have raised glucose or who are at increased risk (e.g. positive family history of diabetes, are obese or have previously had gestational diabetes) should be offered a glucose tolerance test.

The importance of gestational diabetes is still the subject of some debate, but mothers with it tend to have bigger babies and perhaps more chance of birth defects.

Treatment of gestational diabetes is first by paying attention to exercise and diet – sometimes that is all that's needed. Regular blood glucose checks are needed to ensure that the levels are not creeping too high, particularly after meals. If so then insulin therapy will be recommended but can be stopped when the baby is born. At the postnatal check some six to eight weeks after the birth another glucose tolerance test can be done to check if impaired glucose tolerance is still present.

Chapter 15

Diabetes in Childhood

The bulk of this book is about diabetes in adults. Diabetes in childhood has many similarities but also many differences. It is a specialised subject in its own right and only some main points are presented here.

90–95 per cent of people under 16 with diabetes have Type 1. It is an uncommon disease but there are marked variations around the world, and even in the UK, in the numbers of children affected. In England and Wales 17 children per 100,000 develop diabetes each year but in Scotland the figure is 25 per 100,000. In Finland the figure is 43 and Japan 3 per 100,000. Three times as many young people with diabetes are being seen now compared to 30 years ago.

In the recent past young children with Type 2 diabetes have been seen for the first time in the USA and Europe, probably in part caused by the increasing trend towards obesity in our society, but this does not explain the increase in the numbers of Type 1 diabetic children who make up the majority of new cases. As with adults the cause of childhood diabetes is not understood but probably involves a combination of genes and environmental triggers. The majority of children who develop Type 1 do not however have a family history of diabetes.

A number of inherited types of diabetes exist that are more commonly seen by specialists in childhood diabetes. They are quite rare and are not covered further here.

Symptoms

The main symptoms of thirst, weight loss, tiredness and frequent urination are the same as in adults and tend to come on over a short period of a few weeks. Symptoms that are more typical for children include tummy pains, headaches or behaviour problems. Sometimes the diagnosis is delayed and a child will reach the stage of ketoacidosis before being detected, but this is less common than it used to be in the UK due to better awareness on the part of the public and health professionals of the signs to look for. Diabetes should be considered in any child with an otherwise unexplained history of malaise or tummy pains for a few weeks, but the vast majority of children with those symptoms will not be diabetic.

When a young person is diagnosed with diabetes they should be referred to the regional specialist in childhood diabetes without delay.

Treatment

The specialised nature of childhood diabetic management means that most children are cared for by the hospital rather than the primary care team, but this does not mean the family practice is unimportant. Quite the reverse, as caring for a child with diabetes is very much a family affair and can only benefit from proper support from the GP and colleagues in the community. Good communication between the hospital and the primary care teams is essential and the best-organised childhood diabetes services do this well. Liaison nurses trained in diabetes and based in the hospital can bridge the gap between the two services.

Insulin treatment applies to almost all diabetic children. Most now use frequent daily dosage regimes of soluble insulin during the day and longer acting doses at night and increasing numbers of older children use continuous insulin pumps.

The goals of good glucose control and avoidance of hypos apply as much or more to children with diabetes as to adults – many of the complications of diabetes increase with the length of time diabetes has been present. Children bring their own problems in relation to diet restrictions, activity levels and compliance with authority and instructions. One of the many skills required by the family and carers of a child with diabetes is the ability to see through difficult times when various parties fail to see eye to eye.

Families can be put under considerable strain when coping with any long-term medical condition and need good access to back-up support. That should be available through the primary care and hospital teams as well as social services when required. Unfortunately such support is not yet evenly available across the country. Useful national contacts and support services are listed in appendix C.

Chapter 16

The Challenge of Diabetes

Challenge to the individual

If you have diabetes or have read this book you will appreciate that it is an important medical condition with potentially serious consequences. Hopefully you will also now know that it is a treatable condition, and that good care of diabetes will minimise the complications. There are many people who have had diabetes for decades and remain in good health.

Nonetheless, the knowledge that you have diabetes can come as a shock. Particularly with Type 2 disease there can be a slow onset and few symptoms for months or even years before the diagnosis is made, so one minute you might feel only vaguely out of sorts and the next minute your doctor is telling you that you have diabetes. Suddenly you could feel that you have a life-threatening illness or at best one that will inevitably cause disability. It's important to put diabetes firmly in its place though. You can take charge of diabetes, and not let it be the other way around.

You will have seen that diet advice in diabetes does not mean remembering endless lists of calorie values of foods – a healthy diet is the same for diabetic and non-diabetic people. True you can't take the same liberties that you could get away with (in the short term) before you became diabetic, but it doesn't mean you can't ever have a treat.

If you need to move on to tablets then they are easy to take and have few side effects when taken properly. Additional treatment to control high blood pressure and/or high cholesterol is a common need with Type 2 diabetes in particular, so more pills might be required for that, but again it should be possible to get a combination that suits you – there are plenty of choices in blood pressure medicine and the 'statin' drugs that are commonly used to lower cholesterol are well tolerated.

Insulin treatment is nothing like as much trouble as it can seem from just reading about it. Speaking to someone who has Type 1 diabetes is a much better way to get to know what it is really like. It's not all about painful injections (they aren't sore at all once you get the hang of them) – it's really about feeling so much better again after getting onto the treatment that you need once you develop Type 1 diabetes, or if your Type 2 condition progresses to the stage where insulin becomes necessary.

You'll have noticed that throughout the book there are various targets to aim for – blood glucose, HbA$_{1c}$, blood pressure, cholesterol, weight, exercise. It might all sound pretty demanding, and what if you can't get to target – does it mean you are bound to be in trouble? Not so. Look at it that every move *towards* a target that you manage to achieve is a positive contribution to your health. If you look at diabetes as a test that you either pass or fail then you will get disappointed every time a glucose reading comes back a bit high. You do have to work at keeping diabetes under control, but it shouldn't become the dominating factor in your life.

Remember that we have a problem with detecting diabetes early, so you could do your bit for others and encourage people you know to be aware of the symptoms. Spread the word about getting checked out for diabetes, and show by your own example that the earlier the diagnosis is made and treatment is started, the sooner you get back to feeling well and staying that way.

Challenge to the health services

When the National Health Service was born in 1948 few people could have foreseen how successful and long lasting the new system would turn out to be. The organisation of general practice into one of local practitioners having lists of patients ensured that, regardless of income, anyone could see a doctor without paying a fee and it allowed continuity of care, which remains one of the most important and valuable parts of the British medical system.

At that time the population's health was seen as a battle largely won. Mortality from common illnesses was a fraction of what it had been a hundred years earlier due to massive improvements in living conditions, water quality, sanitation and food supply. The advent of antibiotics in the 1940s seemed to herald an age in which medical advance would wipe out all illness. The focus however was very much on the treatment of illness within hospitals. By contrast, general practice was the unglamorous face of medicine, usually looked down upon by specialists and shunned by the best medical graduates who were attracted to brighter lights and higher rewards.

Those attitudes have changed and primary care is now seen in its proper light as the only setting in which the biggest challenge – improving the health of the population – can occur. Unfortunately we still have an organisational structure within primary care that has hardly changed in half a century – and much of the way GPs are organised and resourced is poorly set up to take on the huge task of population-based health improvement.

It is not difficult to be critical too of the influence politicians have had upon the NHS. The diabetes 'epidemic' for example has not happened overnight. It has been seen coming for at least 20 years, yet the last two decades of the twentieth century were characterised by politically driven fragmentation of the health service instead of building a structure of co-operation that we now find ourselves struggling to achieve.

This however is not a book about politics. We need to accept that as we stand we have a major problem on our hands and we need to tackle it. There is much to be commended in the present government moves to improve major health issues such as diabetes.

The National Service Framework for diabetes is the set of goals and quality standards, put forward in December 2001 by the government, that need to be met in dealing with diabetes in England and Wales. The equivalent document in Scotland is the Scottish Framework for diabetes (internet links to both are listed in appendix A). At the time of writing (July 2002) the final parts of these documents are due for publication and are eagerly awaited – they will detail the resources that will be provided to meet the targets that we know have to be achieved.

Many doctors are concerned that not only will there be a shortfall in resources, but also that the targets themselves are unachievable. They feel that to get blood pressure, glucose and cholesterol readings down to target levels we will have huge numbers of patients taking vast amounts of drugs. Perhaps there is some truth in this anxiety but to accept it completely is both defeatist and flies in the face of what are now very solid facts concerning diabetes and these other health issues. We know what the targets are and what we need to do is move towards them, even if actually reaching them is a difficult and perhaps impossible goal for everyone.

Central to achieving any worthwhile targets is the support and encouragement of the public. It will be expensive to fund the health service to the sort of level that will have an impact on major health problems like diabetes, and that money has to come largely from taxation. Even more important is the role of the individual in improving the lifestyle factors that are so important in diabetes, high blood pressure, coronary heart disease and so on. No doctor can make someone change his or her way of living – it has to come from the person concerned.

First, though, one has to know why it is important to act in certain ways. We hope very much that this book has given you the necessary information to understand the reasons behind the recommendations for managing diabetes. We also hope that not only will you apply them to yourself but that you will encourage the 'powers that be' to make the right moves to properly deal with this major national health hazard.

Appendix A

References

Definitions

- American Diabetes Association, 'Report of the expert committee on the diagnosis and classification of diabetes mellitus' (Diabetes Care, 1997; 20: 1183–97).
- Wareham, N.J., and O'Rahilly, S., 'The changing classification and diagnosis of diabetes' (British Medical Journal, 1998; 317: 359–60); http://bmj.com/cgi/content/full/317/7155/359

Causes

- Thorsdottir, I., et al., 'Different beta-casein fractions in Icelandic versus Scandinavian cows' milk may influence diabetogenicity of cows' milk in infancy and explain low incidence of insulin-dependent diabetes mellitus in Iceland' (Pediatrics, 2000: 106 (4): 719–24);

http://www.ncbi.nlm.nih.gov/entrez/query.fcgi?cmd=
Retrieve&db=PubMed&list_uids=11015514&dopt=Abstract

Research studies

- United Kingdom Prospective Diabetes Study Group (UKPDS); http:/
  /www.dtu.ox.ac.uk/index.html?maindoc=/ukpds/
- Diabetes Control and Complications Trial (DCCT); http://content.
  nejm.org/cgi/content/full/329/14/977

Lifestyle intervention

- Diabetes Prevention Programme (DPP), 'Reduction in the incidence
  of Type 2 diabetes with lifestyle intervention or metformin' (New
  England Journal of Medicine, 2002; 346: 393–403); http://content.
  nejm.org/cgi/content/abstract/346/6/393
- Tuomilehto, J,. et al., 'Prevention of type 2 diabetes mellitus by
  changes in lifestyle among subjects with impaired glucose tolerance'
  (New England Journal of Medicine, 2001; 344: 1343–50); http://
  content.nejm.org/cgi/content/full/344/18/1343

Complications of diabetes

- Beach, K.W., et al., 'Progression of lower extremity arterial occlusive
  disease in Type 2 diabetes mellitus' (Diabetes Care, 1988; 11: 464–
  720).
- Preservation of sight in diabetes: a risk reduction programme;
  www.diabetic-retinopathy.screening.nhs.uk/diabetic-retinopathy.
  html
- Parving, I., et al., 'The effect of irbesartan on the development of
  diabetic nephropathy in patients with type 2 diabetes' (New England
  Journal of Medicine, 2001; 345: 870–8); http://content.nejm.org/cgi/
  content/abstract/345/12/870

Guidelines and standards of care

- 'Management of diabetes: a national clinical guideline' (Scottish Intercollegiate Guidelines Network (SIGN), number 55, November 2001); http://www.sign.ac.uk/guidelines/fulltext/55/index.html
- National Service Framework for diabetes; http://www.doh.gov.uk/nsf/diabetes/index.htm
- Scottish Framework for Diabetes; http://www.show.scot.nhs.uk/crag/topics/diabetes/fwork/sdf01.htm
- National Institute for Clinical Excellence (NICE); http://www.nice.org.uk/cat.asp?cn=toplevel

Childhood diabetes

- Greene, S., 'Diabetes in Childhood and Adolescence' (Medicine, 2002; 30: 60–5).

Appendix B

Diabetes Drug Therapy (class examples)

Only brief details of each drug are given here. Full details are included in the manufacturer's data sheets and can also be viewed within the medicines section of the NetDoctor web site http://www.netdoctor. co.uk/medicines/

The information is accurate at the time of writing but new information on medicines appears regularly. A health professional should always be consulted concerning the prescription and use of medicines.

Medicines and their possible side effects can affect individual people in different ways. The following lists some of the side effects that are known to be associated with these medicines. Side effects other than those listed may exist.

A. Insulins in current use

Speed of action	Brand name	Manufacturer	Source or type A = animal H = human sequence
Very quick	NovoRapid (insulin aspart)	Novo Nordisk	H
	Humalog (insulin lispro)	Lilly	H
Quick (soluble insulin)	Hypurin bovine & porcine Neutral	CP	A
	Actrapid	Novo Nordisk	Both available
	Human Velosulin	Novo Nordisk	H
	Humulin S	Lilly	H
	Insuman Rapid	Aventis	H
Intermediate (NPH/isophane insulin and lente insulin)	Hypurin bovine & porcine isophane and lente	CP	A
	Insulatard	Novo Nordisk	Both available
	Humulin I	Lilly	H
	Insuman Basal	Aventis	H
	Human Monotard	Novo Nordisk	H
	Humulin Lente	Lilly	H
Long acting (ultralente insulin)	Human Ultratard	Novo Nordisk	H
	Humulin Zn	Lilly	H
	Insulin glargine (available in UK August 2002)	Aventis	H
Very long acting (protamine zinc insulin)	Hypurin Bovine PZI	CP	A

Biphasic (mixed) insulins		
Brand name	Manufacturer	Source or type A = animal H = Human sequence
Humalog Mix 25 & Mix50	Lilly	H
Humulin M2, M3 & M5		
Human Mixtard 10,20,30, 40 & 50	Novo Nordisk	H
NovoMix 30		
Pork Mixtard 30		A
Insuman Comb 15, 25 & 50	Aventis	H
Hypurin Porcine 30/70 Mix	CP	A

B. Oral hypoglycaemic drugs

In this section an example drug from each category is listed.

1 DRUGS THAT REDUCE INSULIN RESISTANCE

Metformin (biguanide)

How does it work?

First, it reduces the amount of sugar produced by cells in the liver. Second, it increases the sensitivity of muscle cells to insulin. Finally, it also delays absorption of sugar from the intestines into the bloodstream after eating. Overall, metformin reduces blood sugar levels both between and directly after meals. Metformin is used as a first line treatment of type 2 diabetes, particularly in overweight people, when diet and exercise have failed to control blood sugar levels. It can also be used in combination with other antidiabetic medicines to provide better control of blood sugar.

Main side effects
- Metallic taste;
- flushing of the skin;

- loss of appetite;
- elevated levels of lactic acid in the blood (lactic acidosis);
- disturbances of the gut such as nausea, vomiting, diarrhoea or abdominal pain.

Proprietary names of medications containing metformin
Glucamet, Glucophage.

Pioglitazone (thiazolidinedione)

How does it work?
Pioglitazone helps to lower blood sugar levels by increasing the sensitivity of liver, fat and muscle cells to insulin. Pioglitazone also reduces the amount of glucose produced by the liver. Pioglitazone is only licensed for people whose blood sugar is not controlled by the maximum doses of either metformin or a sulphonylurea such as gliclazide and is taken in addition to the other oral antidiabetic medicine.

Main side effects
- Headache;
- excess wind in the digestive system (flatulence);
- inability of a man to have an erection (impotence);
- weight gain;
- visual disturbances;
- dizziness;
- low red blood cell count (anaemia);
- pain in the joints;
- blood in the urine;
- excessive fluid retention (more likely if taken with non-steroidal anti-inflammatory medicines).

Proprietary name of pioglitazone
Actos.

2 DRUGS THAT INCREASE THE RELEASE OF INSULIN FROM THE PANCREAS

Gliclazide (sulphonylurea)

How does it work?
Gliclazide increases the release of insulin from the beta cells of the pancreas. It improves insulin production immediately after eating. This is called early or first phase insulin secretion, and does not normally happen in people with type 2 diabetes. The enhanced insulin production results in a blood sugar lowering effect in response to meals or glucose, as occurs naturally in non-diabetic people.

Gliclazide has been shown to prevent blood cells called platelets from clumping together in the blood. It also increases the breakdown of blood clots that form within the blood vessels. This may help prevent the long-term complications of diabetes, which may be partly due to changes in the blood vessels caused by these mechanisms.

Main side effects
- Low blood glucose level (hypoglycaemia);
- indigestion
- liver disorders;
- blood disorders;
- skin rashes;
- disturbances of the gut such as diarrhoea, constipation, nausea, vomiting or abdominal pain;
- gliclazide may alter the anti blood-clotting effects of warfarin and other anticoagulants.

The following medicines may enhance the blood sugar lowering effect of gliclazide. This may cause unpredictable hypoglycaemia:

- ACE inhibitors, e.g. captopril, enalapril;
- anticoagulants, e.g. warfarin;

- antifungal medicines, e.g. miconazole (miconazole should not be taken with gliclazide);
- large doses of aspirin;
- beta-blockers, e.g. atenolol;
- cimetidine;
- disopyramide;
- monoamine oxidase inhibitor (MAOI) antidepressants, e.g. phenelzine;
- non-steroidal anti-inflammatory drugs (NSAIDs), e.g. ibuprofen;
- tetracycline antibiotics, e.g. oxytetracycline, doxycycline.

Proprietary names of medications containing gliclazide
Diaglyk, Diamicron, Vivazide.

Repaglinide (meglitinide)

How does it work?
Repaglinide increases the amount of insulin released from the pancreas. It works very quickly and is therefore taken just before a meal. Repaglinide may be used alone or in addition to other antidiabetic medications.

Main side effects
- Abdominal pain;
- constipation;
- diarrhoea;
- allergy to the active ingredients, including rash;
- Alteration in results of liver function tests;
- nausea and vomiting.

The following medications may increase the effects of repaglinide and cause low blood sugar levels:

- antibiotics (rifampicin, erythromycin);
- antifungal drugs (fluconazole, itraconazole, ketoconazole).

Proprietary name of repaglinide
NovoNorm.

3 DRUG THAT SLOWS CARBOHYDRATE DIGESTION

Acarbose (alpha glucosidase inhibitor)

How does it work?

Alpha glucosidase is an enzyme present in the lining of the gut that breaks down complex carbohydrates such as starches into molecules small enough for absorption. A carbose inhibits the activity of this enzyme and therefore slows down the digestion and absorption of carbohydrates from the gut. This reduces the normal rise in blood sugar following a meal, and the daily fluctuations in blood sugar are smoothed out. Consequently if a hypoglycaemic attack occurs during treatment with acarbose, it should be treated with glucose not sucrose (cane sugar), as acarbose will delay the absorption of sucrose.

Main side effects

- Excess wind in the stomach and intestines (flatulence);
- abdominal pain;
- diarrhoea;
- rash;
- alteration in results of liver function tests;
- acarbose may alter digoxin levels, and these should therefore be monitored if acarbose is used with digoxin.

Proprietary name of acarbose

Glucobay.

Appendix C

Contacts and Information

Diabetes UK

Diabetes UK is the leading charity working for people with diabetes.
Its website is: www.diabetes.org.uk/home.htm

REGIONAL OFFICES

London
10 Parkway
London NW1 7AA
Tel: 020 7424 1000
Fax: 020 7424 1001

Northern & Yorkshire
Birch House
80 Eastmount Road
Darlington DL1 1LE
Tel:01325 488606
Fax: 01325 488816

North-West
65 Bewsey Street
Warrington WA2 7JQ
Tel: 01925 653281
Fax: 01925 653288

West Midlands
1 Eldon Court
Eldon Street
Walsall WS1 2JP
Tel:01922 614500
Fax: 01922 646789

Northern Ireland
John Gibson House
257 Lisburn Road
Belfast BT9 7EN
Tel: 028 9066 6646
Fax: 028 9066 6333

Scotland
Savoy House
140 Sauchiehall Street
Glasgow G2 3DH
Tel: 0141 332 2700
Fax: 0141 332 4880

Wales
Quebec House
Castlebridge
Cowbridge Road East
Cardiff CF11 9AB
Tel: 029 2066 8276
Fax: 029 2066 8329

Diabetes Research & Wellness Foundation

The Diabetes Research & Wellness Foundation is an organisation of
diabetes patients, their parents and their friends who join together in a
'Diabetes Wellness Network' to help all those afflicted by diabetes.

Office 101/102
Northney Marina
Hayling Island
Hampshire PO11 0NH
Tel: 023 9263 7808 (Administration and Enquiries)
Tel: 023 9263 6132 (Publications)
Fax: 023 9263 6137
Website: www.diabeteswellnessnet.org.uk/

Diabetes Scotland

The aim of this website is to bring together information about a variety
of centres and initiatives that are working together to improve the care
of children with diabetes in Scotland and beyond.

Website: www.diabetes-scotland.org/

Juvenile Diabetes Research Foundation

JDRF funds research into diabetes and disseminates information about diabetes and research progress through publications and public meetings.

19 Angel Gate
City Road
London EC1V 2PT
Tel: 020 7713 2030
Fax: 020 7713 2031

International Diabetes Federation

Website: www.idf.org/home/

Moorfields Eye Hospital

This hospital is one of the main centres for eye disease treatment in the UK, with an international reputation. The Moorfields website contains much useful information on all eye diseases, including diabetic retinopathy.

Website: www.moorfields.org.uk/EyeHealth/DiabeticRetinopathy